"So many people don't even realize they feel worthless. That's when we are in active addiction. Nate breaks it down for you and shows you how he was able to become worthy to the world . . . but mostly to himself. A must read."

—Ken Seeley, CCMI-M, CIP, CTP
Founder , Intervention 911

"Nathan takes us on a very heartfelt and humbling journey into the dark abyss of alcoholism. He then introduces us to the light of recovery and his newfound way of living. The courage to tell his story in such an open forum and expose his life to all of us is remarkable and an invaluable gift. To witness his complete transformation is both a blessing and a tremendous message of hope. His "Recovery Roots" provide powerful guideposts that enhance the path of life for all. He is a man that has earned a serene spot in bright sunshine. May we all learn from his experience and wisdom and join him on this journey of life!"

—Dave Beck, CPA
Cirque Lodge Director of Experiential Therapies

"Whenever I think of Nathan Kruse, the same two words come to mind: joy and gratitude. Nate exudes both in spades, but that wasn't always his way. "Nate, the Early Years," was fear-based and trauma filled with some challenging troubles thrown in. But in December 2012 when we met, Nate was ON FIRE with recovery. He'd found his first spec of sobriety and humility and was seeking sanity in his surrender. He was a work in progress, and working he was. Initially,

"I didn't see Nate's pain because he was living his life in a new found freedom and reveling in it. The smile in his eyes was the first thing I noticed about him as it was vibrant and full of hope. It still is today. Recovery Rx is a demonstration of the hard work and healing Nate has achieved in eight short years. He crawled into treatment an open, oozing wound *and today he has a life he and many others are proud of. He's living the promises with his sweetheart and sweet baby girl. By the way, I enjoyed his book too!"*

—Jamie Eater, MSW, MAC, CAP, CIP, CTT
Executive Director, Sober Escorts, Inc.

"Recovery Rx provides a rare opportunity to look behind the curtain; to view a family that, on the outside, appears wealthy, attractive, and extremely successful. However, behind this sturdy facade, you will find a crumbling family, suffering greatly, wounding each other deeply, and on a tragic trajectory. Yet, from the bitter seeds of childhood neglect and abuse now grows a strong confident man. I am Nate's proud mother. This book validates this truth; with the right recovery tools, all past suffering can indeed be transformed into a brilliant, successful, and meaningful life. Recovery Rx is perfect for both individuals and family members caught in the vicious vortex of addiction."

— Caroline Smith, MA, LPC, CSAT
Director of Addiction Services & Intensive Workshops
Pine Grove Behavioral Health

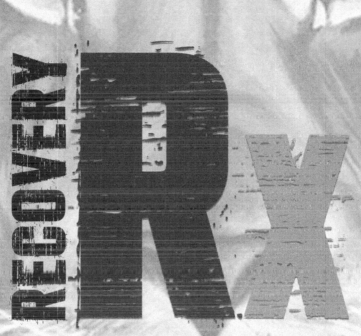

"Nathan takes us on a heartfelt and humbling journey
into the dark abyss of alcoholism;
then introduces us to the light of recovery."
—Dave Beck, Cirque Lodge Director

RECOVERY RX

From Worthless to Worthy

Nathan Kruse

Recovery Rx
From Worthless to Worthy

Nathan Kruse

© Copyright 2020 Nathan Kruse

All rights reserved.

BookWise Publishing
www.BookWisePublishing.com
chrisbizzz@comcast.net

Book Design by K Christoffersen
Lion illustration by Darshonna Lieberman,
www.darshonna.com
iStock background by Allusioni
The Flast font by Quirino Sosas/Knapsack Studio

Library of Congress Control Number: 2020909611
Nathan Kruse
Recovery Rx /Kruse, Nathan

ISBN 978-1-60645-257-8 Paperback $14.99
ISBN 978-1-60645-253-0 eBook $9.99
ISBN 978-1-60645-254-7 Audio $19.99

10 9 8 7 6 5 4 3 2 1

7/26/2020

www.TheRecoveryRx.com
Facebook.com/Recovery-Rx
RecoveryRx.podbean.com

TABLE OF CONTENTS

Dedication ix

Preface... xi

Foreword... xv

1 1

2 5

3 9

4 11

5 15

6 33

7 37

8 45

9 53

10 57

11 63

12 65

13 69

14 75

15 79

16 83

17 89

18 93

19 85

20 99

21 109

22 119

23 123

24 127

25 137

26 143

27 157

28 165

My Recovery Roots 167

Postscript 197

Acknowledgments 207

About the Author 211

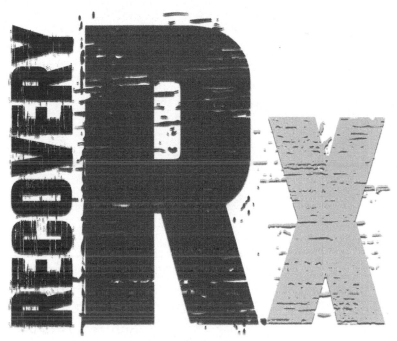

From Worthless to Worthy

Nathan Kruse

Sobriety is never owned. It's rented, and rent is due every day.

DEDICATION

I dedicate this book to those who are still suffering as alcoholics and addicts, not to forget the family members and those suffering from mental illnesses, to whom this book applies as well. May you find your Higher Power and take comfort knowing it is never too late to save yourself.

I also dedicate this book to all of the amazing people who work in the Recovery field. With your tireless efforts and passion, you give us hope and the skills to create a life of abundance.

—Nathan Kruse

*Recovery is literally
to recapture
and reclaim
that which has been
lost or stolen.*

—Caroline Smith

PREFACE

I'm Nathan Kruse, and I'm a grateful recovering alcoholic and addict. I wasn't always this way as you will find out in my book.

In my adolescent years I felt useless and forgotten as I grew up. Then, in my early adult life I *became* worthless to the ones around me, and most importantly to myself. I pushed all of these negative and adverse feelings deep within me with the assistance of copious amounts of alcohol.

It wasn't until after years of drinking away my problems that I realized the problems were only getting bigger; I knew I was screwed.

I have honored my burning desire to share my story of certain death due to alcoholism to finding and cultivating a thriving Recovery program I put in practice every day. I named this book *Recovery Rx* because I am completely rooted in Recovery and want to share what I call my 10 Recovery Roots with you. These 10 roots are practical applications that can be used in any form of sobriety and wellness to overcome damaging triggers, life's curve balls, and self-sabotaging. I call it a prescription of freedom, but you must do the work to achieve it.

For the past four years of my life, I have worked to complete this book hoping it will inspire you, the reader. It started as a dream, but it hasn't always been a dream to write it. I've had to relive the worst times in my life to uncover my disease of addiction. But it's also been very gratifying to see how far I have come from death's doorstep. I believe everything is in God's timing, and over these past four years I have grown in my Recovery and developed new ways to stay sober and live in an abundance of gratitude. I now have the opportunity to support my brothers and sisters in Recovery. By giving back my time, I am able to keep my sobriety front and center. Thank you for joining me on this journey and enjoy the ride.

With much love and mindfulness,
Nate

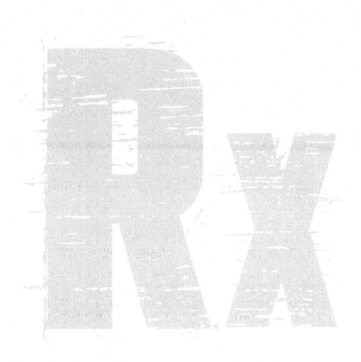

*"Only you
can make a
difference in your life.*
—Nathan Kruse

FOREWORD

'm allergic to alcohol. My whole body is drawn to it. But the simple fact is, to me it's poison. Now, more than eight years sober, I still refuse to kid myself. I'm an alcoholic. I always will be, even if I never take another drink for the rest of my life. Alcohol dependence is a chronic medical disease. I know that when I drink, I cannot stop like other people. Knowing this has saved my life and continues to save it every day since it all began.

RX

The first time I drank hard liquor, it burned, but in a good way, like those cinnamon bear candies Grandma gave us when we stayed with her. She let us have one a day, like a vitamin. Sometimes I'd chew it to feel the heat explode in my mouth. Other times I'd let it sit on my tongue. It burned, but I liked controlling how much it hurt, and how fast it stopped hurting. A lot of stuff hurt when I was a kid, and I couldn't stop them from happening. I didn't mind making my mouth burn because I knew I could control that.

Controlling pain, numbing myself to reality—anything that distanced me from it, I was up for it. That's probably why I loved getting drunk so much. It was my way of escaping the real shit that seemed to be attracted to me like those tiny lead and metal filings in the dirt as I dragged a magnet through it when I was a kid. My painted-red U-shaped magnet collected

them like crazy. Remember those days? The most carefree of
my life, and yet . . . not.

Everything is different now, because I'm sober. Sobriety has given me many gifts. One of the biggest is of feeling
deeply again. I used to feel a lot when I was a kid. I think
these emotions contributed significantly to the eventual development of my disease: I felt too much—too much discom-
fort. I think that's what got me addicted in the first place:
I felt too much. Now I can't get enough: good feelings, bad
feelings, and everything in between. It's all good because it's
real and happening the way it's supposed to. Some people call
it fate; I call it God, and I am so grateful to be on this journey
with Him. After my daughter was born, I really understood
gratitude. When the baby and her mother were safe, I had a
flood of gratitude, this powerful rush of feeling. I hadn't felt
anything like that in a long time, maybe ever. That was a big
change in me. Before Josie was born, I had to actively look for
things to be grateful for. Now I just look at her, and I understand joy on a new level.

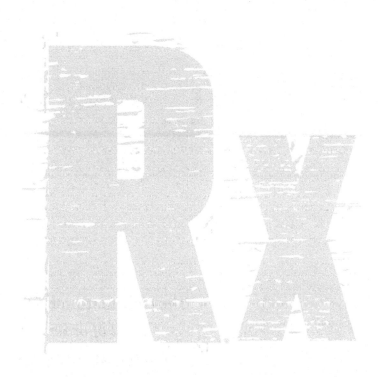

*The elevator to sobriety
is out of order.
You must use the steps.*

1

My parents, Tom and Caroline met at a Midwestern University during the early 70s. He was a charismatic junior and she was a naive freshman. They were engaged one month after meeting and married within ten months. Upon the end of her freshman year, my mom left college. Interestingly, my dad had a fake graduation. He participated in the university's graduation ceremony, wore the ceremonial cap and gown, and accepted congratulations and gifts. The Dean allowed Tom to attend the ceremony on the condition that he would rapidly complete the three credit hours needed for his degree. Even after receiving this gracious extension, Tom never finished college or received his diploma. He told no one, not even my mother. During his professional career, he fraudulently claimed to have an undergraduate degree. Upon his "graduation," and while still living in Illinois, my brother Blaine was born. The family moved two more times prior to my birth.

Following Blane's birth by two and a half years, on a hot muggy July day in 1977, I arrived on the scene in the capital city of Lincoln, Nebraska. Jimmy Carter had been sworn in as the 39th President of the US and immediately began pardoning Viet Nam draft evaders. Rent was cheap. Gas cost 65 cents a gallon. You could get a very decent three bedroom/two bath home for around $33,000. And the King of Rock and Roll died at the young age of 42. Bummer.

But some other really great things came on the scene too. For example, the first, and may I say one of the greatest, game systems, Atari 2600, made its appearance. Steve Jobs came up with the Apple II, and, as I already mentioned, I arrived on the scene. The cost for me, a little over $2,000, slightly pricier than the Apple II, but I was worth every penny. Oh, I failed to mention that just two months before I was delivered, George Lucas delivered as well. *Star Wars* opened in theaters in May 1977.

In terms of delivery, my mom and Tom seemed pretty happy to have added a second son to the Kruse family. Blaine, a toddler now, allowed himself to be replaced as the "baby." I don't think Mom had a clue about the destructive future ahead of us. Tom was gone a lot, money was scarce, and she had her hands full with two highly energized boys. During this time both of my parents began amassing their emotional ammo for their own "star wars" ahead.

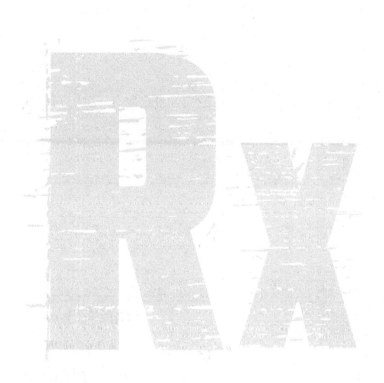

*There are only
two options:
make progress
or make excuses.*

2

Caroline's relationship with Tom was anything but safe, but she had difficulty acknowledging the danger. The grave adversity she experienced during her childhood significantly impaired her ability to protect, honor, value, or even enjoy her true self. This is only one example of Caroline's impairment.

This incident happened while my parents were dating and would have been a red flag for most women. While holding hands, Tom and Caroline were walking across the center of campus as a buxom blond walked toward them. Upon seeing this other woman, Tom immediately dropped Caroline's hand and proceeded to speak flirtatiously with *Miss Buxom*. Rather than question Tom's abrupt and disrespectful behavior, Caroline compared herself to this other woman, found herself to be lacking, and therefore, lucky to be engaged to Tom. That's how callous he could be and how insecure Caroline was.

Their destructive dance of his arrogant avoidance and her insecure anxiety only grew worse after they married. Believing it was her duty to make Tom happy, Caroline minimized, rationalized, and justified his frequent demeaning behaviors and shaming words. Unfortunately, the expenditure of effort to please a person who simply wouldn't be pleased came at a high price; her soul started to shrivel and her energy wane.

Following Blane's birth, the family moved to Michigan where Tom had accepted a job as a youth pastor. Mom was 21 at the time and became pregnant with me within months of arriving in Michigan. Tom was gone a lot overseeing youth activities and Caroline was a proud minister's wife.

After less than twelve months in his position, one of Tom's dirty secrets detonated. Out of the blue, Tom came home and told Caroline he had just resigned his position and they would have to move. Shell-shocked and trying to desperately to understand, Caroline begged Tom to tell her why he had quit. Tom said that after praying about it, he just didn't feel the ministry was for him. But the truth eventually came out; Tom had been fired.

What actually occurred was a shocking validation that the ministry certainly wasn't for him. Apparently, church leadership had received several complaints about Tom's sexualizing and flirtatious behaviors. With no job prospects, little savings, a pregnant wife, and small toddler, Tom accepted a job with my mom's dad. My grandfather had a construction business in Lincoln and agreed to let Tom work for him.

Upon their move to Nebraska, I was born with such bad jaundice that I had to stay in the hospital after my mother was discharged. These were the days before they let you stay overnight with a sick baby, so Mom had to leave me there. Every day, she dropped Blaine off with Grandma and came to the hospital. This went on for a week, and it was during this time that Tom said something so bad to my grandfather that he fired him. To this day, no one knows what Tom said.

My Granddad was so furious that he forbade my grandmother from having anything to do with Tom, including her own daughter! So there was Mom, suffering from postpartum depression, with a toddler, a sickly newborn, no car, no friends, no support, no money, and no idea why her father was punishing her for something Tom had done. But that was my grandfather: he ruled Grandma, and, in so doing, he ruled my mom as well.

It was a torturous, horrible time. We didn't even have enough money to buy food. Mom called the Red Cross to see if they would buy her blood, but they refused because of my recent birth. Meanwhile, her depression worsened and, to survive, she turned inward and away from her young sons. She went through the usual routines, bathing us, dressing us, and feeding us as best she could, but she was in no way fully present.

Mom said I got the worst of it because I spent the first week of my life in the hospital and my early months with a mother who was too depressed and forlorn to make me feel seen, soothed, or safe. She didn't know how to do that for herself, and as she still says, "To my everlasting sorrow, I couldn't do it for my two beautiful sons."

*Old keys
won't open
new doors.*

3

In early 1982, when I was five years old, our family moved to southern California. Tom had found employment with a company that provided financial planning for military officers.

We lived in a modest apartment surrounded by huge oak trees. I was unaware of it at the time, but I had a serious allergic reaction to poison oak and poison ivy and it was everywhere! When we were playing, Blaine and I walked through it or rubbed up against it and I caught some really bad cases of it. I would be home covered in pink calamine lotion just trying not to scratch my skin off.

When I wasn't itching, we went to the shores in Long Beach quite a bit. We would always get a big bucket of Colonel Sanders' Kentucky Fried Chicken, the best chicken on the planet. After we had eaten our fill, we'd feed the beach birds the rest. It was so much fun just playing in the sand and getting kissed by the California sun. These were certainly carefree days.

4

"No one
is ever too lost
to be saved.

4

Tom's success with the company continued to grow, so much so that they sent him to open an office in Sacramento, which meant we headed north for the next three years. This was about the time of the Gulf War which only escalated the need for life insurance and retirement preparations.

I liked Sacramento. It was a city surrounded with some great country, kind of wild, but full of things to explore. We bought our first home and it was amazing. Blaine and I had our own bedrooms, and I, of course, put up my Arnold Schwarzenegger *Commando* movie poster. He was my favorite action hero, and I loved all his movies—*The Predator* and *Twins* to name a few. Oh, don't forget *The Terminator!* We lived in a community called Gold River, where many beautiful homes were being built all along the hillsides.

During this time our family had a lot of fun. Sometimes we'd load up our bikes and take them on trails through the mountains. One time Mom and I were riding under a canopy of trees and happened upon a silkworm infestation. They were so thick; all you could see were silky webs. They would spin down, littering entire trails; but they were hard to see until you were right up on them. Suddenly we rode into a curtain of gross webs. I found that I could duck under the silk, but Mom kept getting slimed and entangled by them! She was screaming bloody murder. I couldn't stop laughing, and it still makes me smile to think about it.

It was perfect to take my Diamondback BMX bike out for long rides with Blaine or even by myself and just get into nature. I found snakes, eagles, and even the occasional bobcat.

We custom-designed a pool and a hot tub in our backyard. It was like a dream; a total oasis for kids. Our family really bonded with swimming, barbecuing, and hiking experiences.

Christmas 1985, my parents bought a Nintendo that just blew my mind. Blaine and I would play videos games like *Zelda*, Mike Tyson's *Punch Out*, *Contra* and, of course, *Mario Bros.*, for hours and hours.

I was seven or eight and Blaine was nine or ten when we were in Sacramento. Life was good but occasionally the odd thing would happen like Tom walking around the house naked. He was a big man, around six feet tall, two hundred and ten pounds and muscular. He was totally inappropriate. Add to that, he made Blaine and me shower with him on Sunday mornings, before church. Any other day of the week, we were allowed to shower alone, but for whatever reason, on Sundays, we had to shower with Tom. He'd stand behind us and soap us up, our entire body, one at a time. I'd go to the end of the tub and sometimes squat, so he'd do Blaine first; then we'd switch places. His privates were at my eye level. I would turn away and not face him because I was so embarrassed, so ashamed. I'd be dying inside. I hated it.

In December 1987, we received word that Tom had received another promotion and that we would be moving to a new place where I didn't want to go—not at all—not in the least. I had been in paradise in northern California, but I had no choice but to move again.

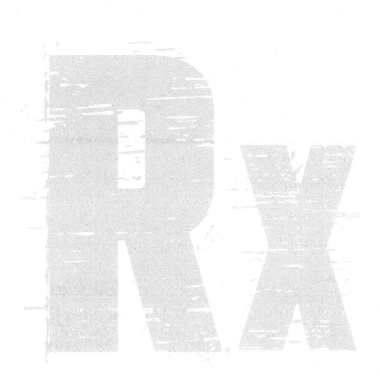

5

*The fears
you don't face
become your
limitations.*

5

ue to his business acumen and success, the company again asked Tom to open a new office in a small town near Frankfurt, Germany. This was 1988; I was eleven years old and spent the next three-and-a-half years in a kind of hell.

My mother had always been very physically active and had created a great social life in California. The beautiful weather, the societal opportunities, entertaining for Tom's associates and management, all contributed to her sense of self-worth and personal fulfillment. But Frankfurt was different; it was one of the grayest, gloomiest places on earth, not to mention the beer capital of the world.

This was where I had my first taste of alcohol, at the ripe young age of eleven. I was with my mom at the tailor's, of all places. The owner was Turkish and he gave patrons chocolates filled with liqueur. In the States, we'd get a mint or something. Not in Germany! He gave my mom one and she took a bite, but when he turned away, she made a face, stuck it in my hand and whispered, "I don't like it—you take it." I ate it and hated it. It tasted nasty.

I don't know how it is now, but at that time in Germany, there was no minimum age for smoking or drinking. At the corner store, you could buy groceries and alcohol, hard liquor, beer, wine, anything. The town where we lived, Altenheim, Baden-Württemberg, was inundated with apple orchards;

they made copious amounts of apple wine. My parents would go away on business trips and my brother would say, "Hey, Nate, go to the store and get a bottle of rum, some whiskey, vodka, and some sodas, and bring it back. We're going to have some friends over." Blaine had gotten to know a few kids at this point, so off I went. And the stores would sell it to me!

On my walk home, I'd have a little taste here and a little taste there. Nothing crazy. I didn't get drunk. Certainly, I didn't know what I was doing; just like when I started smoking and wasn't inhaling. I was just trying to be cool.

Upon arriving in Germany, we rented a huge traditional home. Not including the master suite, Blaine got the best room; mine was horrible. I hated Germany for many reasons, but living in the "spider room" was at the top of the list. I'd go to put my shoes on in the morning and spiders would crawl out, wander up my legs, and out of the sleeves of my shirt. I cried every night, but my parents wouldn't let me sleep with Blaine; that was my room and I had to stay in it.

We were enrolled in a regular school where everyone spoke only German. I don't know what Mom and Tom were thinking; my mom thought that since we were young, we'd just pick up the language. Well, you don't just pick up a language in two weeks, no matter how young you are. Before we left California, my dad hired a German-speaking live-in nanny to move with us and teach Blaine and me the German language. One day during our lessons, we looked out the window and it was snowing; big huge flakes. Blaine and I went crazy—we'd been living in California and had never seen snow before—but this woman wouldn't let us turn around and watch it. We had to sit with our backs to the window, our eyes on her. She only lasted a few months before my mom begged my dad to let her go.

One morning, I was walking to school alone in the dark. There was a butcher shop on the way and on this particular day the doors were open partway. Deep red blood was everywhere, running out the door into the gutter and over the cobblestones. I'd never seen that much blood before, and it scared the hell out of me. Then, peering inside the doors, I saw these two men in long white aprons covered with blood, stirring a vat of water, boiling a pig alive. The pig was jumping, gyrating, squealing, screaming—and there were other animals on the table that were being cut up. The blood was flowing into the street. It was like a horror movie you don't want to see but you can't stop watching. I didn't want it to be real, but I knew it was real, and I didn't know what to do except keep on walking. I wish I could forget it, but I can't. It was horrible.

I didn't tell anyone about the pig; there was no one to tell, really. Blaine was often out with his friends; Tom didn't return from work until ten, and Mom was wiped out, depressed, and in bed.

After living there for about a year, my dad invited one of his past employees and his wife to move from California to Germany. Kevin and Beth accepted his offer and came to live with us. My mom thought having them there would make things better, and in some ways it did, but there were issues. For starters, against Mom's wishes, Tom gave them the master bedroom, and they moved to a smaller bedroom

Another good thing happened during this time; my mom secured a civilian job working for the Air Force. Her position included military ID cards allowing us access to American military bases and commissary shopping. I hated German food, so being able to get American food like *Captain Crunch*, hot dogs or pizza was great. I could go to the base arcade, eat nachos, drink *Coke* and play video games for hours after school. It was a mini-America. I'd finally found a tiny piece of heaven.

But some weird stuff happened too. Like the time Kevin and Tom got the idea that we should all drive up to the Fulda Gap (Fulda-Lücke in German) which was the site of World War II's Battle of the Bulge. Like most hostile countries, East and West Germany had a barrier between them called no man's land. This was 1988 and the Berlin Wall hadn't come down yet so things were still quite hostile between East and West. All six of us piled into Tom's Mercedes and drove the several hours to the Gap. As we approached, I noticed in the distance a massive dark tower on the East German side. The closer we got I could see it was a watchtower, a really high structure with blacked-out windows, protected behind a serious twelve-foot high fence-like wall made of thick iron bars.

Once we exited the car, Kevin said, "Anyone gotta piss? Let's go piss on the wall."

Absolutely! Blaine and I were ready!

Not knowing the danger of what we were about to do, my mom, Beth, and Tom walked away toward a river in the distance. Ignoring the posted red and black *verboten* signs, Kevin led Blaine and me into no-man's land. We unzipped our pants and started peeing through the bars onto East Germany, essentially desecrating their country. Looking around, I relieved myself, I noticed the decaying bodies of dead rabbits and squirrels everywhere. I asked Kevin what they were doing there. He said, "That's what they use for target practice from the watchtower." I was thinking, *These animals are just feet away from us. Could we be shot?*

Next thing you know, sirens were blaring and the West German police came roaring up in this huge van. Like a SWAT Team, several gigantic officers attired fully in black, faces concealed by masks, rushed toward us. As the swarm neared, I noticed their black assault rifles aimed directly at us. They encircled Kevin, Blaine, and me and screamed words we couldn't understand.

All this commotion got my parents attention and they began running back. The police officers immediately arrested all six of us, placed us in handcuffs, and confiscated our American passports. We were forcefully placed into their van and driven to the police station. One of the officers followed us driving Tom's car. Later we learned that the East German police in the watchtower had contacted the West German authorities warning them of our actions and stating that due to our trespass they had the authority to shoot us without recourse or apology.

We were held captive for hours wondering what would happen next. Eventually an English-speaking officer arrived and let us know that our passports would not be returned and therefore we would be deported. But that didn't happen. Evidently Kevin and Tom must have concocted a creative story because the West German police eventually released us, and a few weeks later the American Consulate returned our passports.

I was stunned, how could a bunch of adults be so reckless? I was eleven years old and Blaine was only thirteen; we could both have been shot. Kevin was an Air Force pilot; how could he not know what a dangerous stunt this would be? We were kids; we trusted the adults in our lives to lead by example and keep us safe. Instead, they behaved like reckless, totally irresponsible children.

This is but one example of the unpredictable adult supervision we had in Germany, which is to say, very little.

Added to our frequent family mayhem, many of the Germans we encountered seemed less than welcoming. One afternoon as our family returned home from running errands, we found ourselves the unfortunate recipients of a spectacular "unwelcome" gift. As we neared our home, I observed a most remarkable sight. The entire road surface directly in front of the house had been covered by massive amounts of shattered glass. It was personal; these shards started right where our property started and ended just past our drive. We had to back down the hill and park the car in front of a neighbor's house. It was scary and shocking. As our family swept up the mess, our neighbors silently watched from their balconies, doorways, and windows. No one offered to help; they just stared at us. It was creepy and so unfair. We hadn't done anything to anyone. So I thought, *Fuck 'em all.*

Tom was making so much money by now, he bought himself a fancy 8 series BMW; it was like a rocket, and we took extravagant vacations—skiing in Switzerland, touring Austria, England, Turkey, Istanbul, Israel and Africa—amazing trips. We looked like a rich, happy American family.

RX

I entered fourth grade having come from a school I loved in California to a neighborhood German school where nothing was familiar, nothing was the same, and I couldn't communicate with anyone.

Blaine had a knack for the language and acclimated pretty well, but not me. Since I had a German mental block, I was doing so poorly in school that my parents tried to move me into the American Department of Defense (DOD) school system but were told it was full. Eventually we were enrolled in the very expensive and exclusive Frankfurt International School. FIS was populated with kids from all over the world. Still, since there weren't many Americans, most did not speak English. The British headmaster was like a typical villain in a kid's book— stern, harsh, and always on the lookout for new way to put me down; frequently demanding my parents attend numerous meetings, all focused on my shortcomings; eventually threatening to kick me out and deport me.

It wasn't until I met a kid from Texas—Tyler—that I finally had a friend, even if Texan wasn't really English, it worked! In fact our relationship worked so well, we had a tendency to get in a lot of trouble.

There was a popular restaurant a block away from our house, and the street would be jammed with parked cars on weekends. One Saturday, I invited him to stay overnight, and when it was dark and the restaurant was busy, we slipped flathead screwdrivers into our pockets and moseyed on down. We weren't interested in the restaurant; we just want to wreak havoc on the Germans' cars.

On our way, aboard our skateboards, Tyler and I vandal-
ized as many as we could: he'd pop off hood ornaments, and I
would walk on the other side scratching the shit out of them.
Never mind that we didn't know who the cars belonged to—
almost certainly not to the broken-glass culprits—but, hey,
they were definitely owned by Germans, and that was good
enough for us. I was probably twelve by then, and if people
were going to trample on my rights, I was going to trample
back.

While I had been having a great time vandalizing property, Mom was sinking farther and farther into a debilitat-
ing depression. The signs were there. She slept a lot. She was
always tired. She had no social life at all now since she didn't
speak the language, she had very little opportunity socially.
No friends. And no pun intended, frankly, the German people were rude. Add to that the weather was cold and gloomy,
and coming from sunny California, seasonal affective dis-
order just made her depression worse.

Tom was gone a lot and working constantly; his long
hours, numerous meetings, and frequent European trav-
el were all inflating his financial success and huge ego but
devastating his personal life. As Mother's despair worsened,
mine was just beginning.

Rx

For fun, we'd go to a swimming pool complex, all four
of us, on the weekends sometimes. My mom bought these
neon-yellow skin-tight swimsuits that were cool to have but
were kind of revealing for a 12-year-old boy at a co-ed pool.

One afternoon as we prepared to go home, Blaine and I
went to the locker room to change into our clothes. It was

huge, tons of lockers lining the walls and a strip of changing rooms down the middle. The changing rooms had doors that didn't go all the way to the ground and locked with a plastic latch on the inside. I heard Blaine leave, but I was still in there, taking my time, when all of a sudden this hand comes up from underneath and unlatched the door, opened it, and this strange man jumped inside the stall with me.

I grabbed my clothes, but before I could get them on, I felt his hand touch my genitals. I pushed past him and ran out of there as fast as I could, flying out of the locker room. I saw my family waiting for me down the hall and ran to them. They said, "Hey, Nate, you took forever. You okay?" I told them I was okay, but I was shaking and panting, but they were already walking out, so I followed them to the car. The drive home felt like it took three weeks. I never said a word to anybody—I didn't even tell my parents or my brother; no one. I had felt such unwarranted shame from that incident that I never even told my mom until a few years ago.

RX

When I was 13, our family went to Kenya on a youth trip set up by the organization my mom worked for. Our goal was to lay pipe and bring fresh water to a Masai tribe living in the bush. It was very rural and rustic. As we set up camp, we dug holes for bathrooms and stuck two-by-fours in the ground with plastic sheeting to separate the boys' and girls' stalls.

The first night there, we were sitting on the ground in this huge tent while someone led us in singing something like *Kumbaya*. Mom was sitting in front of me. The tent was dimly lit with only one bulb hanging down in the middle of it. It was so dark it was it black outside and that one bulb attracted huge swarms of insects. Some of these insects were bigger than I'd known were even possible. I was bored and yanked up a clod of dry grass and earth. I thought it would be funny to pitch it at my mom, so I flipped it in the air, and it landed on her leg. Bad move. When it landed, I whispered to her that a big spider had just landed on her. She looked down and in shock tried to brush it off, but the dry roots just clung to the thin fabric of her pants. Unable to rapidly rid herself of the monster, she jumped up, screaming and stamping her feet on the ground. She was so upset she started to cry.

Everything stopped—the music, the singing—and everyone was staring at her. Some of the other adults came over to take her outside, and I went too, patting her on the back and asking if she was okay. She was shaking and crying uncontrollably. It took her a while to calm down. The whole time I was trying to comfort her, I felt like a piece of crap. It was two years before I could tell her that it was me, and I meant it as a joke because we both hate bugs; except it was hard to see in there and she thought it was real. I told her how sorry I was about the whole practical joke, and she laughed hysterically, which is what I love about her: she always forgave me, no matter what.

Rx

Sometimes it seemed like I grew up with few people respecting my rights, so I didn't always respect other people's rights either. During the summer, Mom and Tom used to send us across the country to stay with grandparents; we would be there for up to six weeks sometimes. One of these times they went on a business trip to Hawaii. I wanted to go too. Blaine and I wanted to go wherever they were going. But they said it would be fun staying with our grandparents and seeing our cousins. We told them we'd rather be with them, but they sent us away anyway. It sucked.

On one of these trips, my parents left Blaine and me with Tom's parents on Whidbey Island, Washington. Grandma and Grandpa Kruse had a wooden house surrounded by an acre or two of land. The house was nice: living room with a fireplace; dining room; and two or three bedrooms in the back with a guest room. It felt secluded and quiet, pine trees everywhere. When I smell pine, I remember those days.

Tom's parents were the strictest, meanest, and coldest hyper-religious people ever. The only thing warm in that house were some old, hard gummy bear candies my grandmother kept in a jar. They were cinnamon bears and were hot; they would burn your mouth, which is why it didn't bother me so much that she said I could only have one.

Grandma was suspicious, frail, and veiny, with white pasty skin, and dark beady eyes. Grandpa was tall and thin. He had a big woodworking shop with every tool known to man. He was in there a lot. I think they were retired, but before that, he was a missionary pastor for a long time. And he had a very controlling, strong will . . . my grandma too. In that house, it was their way or the highway; and the highway often hurt.

RX

But I thought, I'm stuck on this frickin' island; I'm going to make friends. There were a few neighborhood boys my age and we'd ride our bikes; we were a bit of a pack. Blaine never came along or made friends with these kids, but I did. We'd shoot hoops in the street and ride our bikes around the neighborhood.

One day one of the kids said, "Hey, some people down the street are out of town. Maybe we could get into their house." I knew this was wrong, no question. But I was bored out of my gourd and I wanted to have some fun. So I said, "Great! Let's try." There were four of us. One kid threw a rock through the back door window; we stuck our hands in, and unlocked the door. We walked in and looked around. I felt uncomfortable and had a strong feeling that I shouldn't be there; I was almost dizzy from the feeling that what I was doing was wrong. But I thought, I'm here, so I'm going through with it. I walked up to the fireplace and someone suggested we start a fire because it was cold. Sure! There was some wood piled up, so we lit it.

When you're a kid, you never think anyone knows anything about what you're doing. But the neighbors knew that the homeowners were away on vacation and wondered why smoke was coming out of the chimney. Meanwhile, we're sitting back, we've got this fire roaring in the fireplace, we're warm, and we're proud of each other for starting a fire. Then we hear sirens. Oh, no!

We jumped up and ran out the back where our bikes were and hauled ass. I rode my bike back to Grandma and Grandpa's as fast as I could and ran inside. They said, " Nate, where've you been?" I remember not answering them and running into the backroom that Blaine and I were sharing, slamming the door, and squeezing down onto the floor between the bed and the wall. The next thing I knew, there was a sharp knocking on the door and my grandfather's very stern voice saying, "Nate, you in there?"

I didn't say anything. Then I heard the door open and, from underneath the bed, I saw these shiny black shoes and black pants with a yellow stripe. It was the cops. They said, "Nate, get out here." Oh, man. I was busted. The cops asked what happened, and I told them we didn't mean anything, we just wanted to be warm, and they listened and told me not to do it again. It was no big deal. That is, until they left. And then I got the beating of my life. It was a belt that time. My Grandpa said, "You're embarrassing me!" That's what he was mad about. I was embarrassing him. His abuse was awful, and I decided I'd do anything to retaliate because he'd beaten me so badly.

But it's not like he never wanted to do anything nice for us, for example, he was in the building mood one day and went out and hung a tire from a rope to make a swing on a huge pine tree in front of the house. Blaine and I would push each other in it. I had a pocket knife, and on this particular day, I retaliated; I took my knife and started sawing at the rope. Grandpa had been watching because he came out of the house and said, "Nate, don't cut that rope." I kept sawing at it, and he told me if I cut the rope and it broke, I would be in a lot of trouble. I just kept sawing until the rope broke and the tire fell on the ground. He went ballistic. He grabbed me by the ear and yanked me hard, kneed me to the ground, dragged me into the house by my ear, threw me in my room, and slammed the door. I was terrified he was going to come back. And then he did and beat me hard with his hand. That hurt, but nothing like the assault and pain he administered to my ear. To this day, I swear my left ear is higher than my right one because he pulled on it so hard.

There's no doubt I was trying to provoke him. He'd gone to some effort to build that swing for Blaine and me, so for me to cut it down right in front of him while he's telling me not to do it—it was an act of rebellion. And I think I know why.

The night before we'd had steaks for dinner the night before which was great, but when I was done and stood up to bring my dish to the sink, he told me to sit back down and finish what was on my plate. There was nothing there but a piece of gristle, a thick, translucent slab of fat, like a hard eyeball. I told him I didn't want to eat it.

"You've got to eat everything," he said.

"But I don't want to eat it! It's gross!"

He stared me down. "You've got to eat it!"

Back and forth it went, with me trying to get out of eating the gristle.

"Well," he said, "you're going to sit here until you eat it."

I tried to swallow it and gagged. I spit it out, and that old man sat there and watched me. The rest of them went to watch TV or sit by the fire or read a book. I had to sit there looking at that nasty knot of gristle. He watched me as I gagged and chewed with saliva running out of my mouth until I got it down. Just thinking about it still makes me nauseous, thirty years later.

RX

Summers in Nebraska with my mother's parents were full of long, hot, muggy days. During this time my grandparents lived in a trailer set up on blocks, as their dream home was being built. Summer temperatures in that trailer almost singed my lungs; it was an oven. Their bedroom was at one end and Blaine and I stayed in the opposite end.

Grandpa was in charge. I had no power, no say-so, no control. I remember episodes of these struggles as if they happened yesterday, even though I was just a kid. They marked me and are impossibly hard to forget.

My grandfather liked to play tricks on me when I was young. Maybe it was the only way he knew how to relate to kids. Trick them and show them how scary life could be before they found out on their own. He was a physically strong guy, burly but lean. He owned his own construction company, worked with cement, steel and rocks, and drove big equipment. He'd take me out on rides in dump trucks and tractors, even taught me how to drive a tractor when I was nine or ten—cool stuff for a kid like me.

One time, I must have been around six or seven, he came into my room really early in the morning and said, "Nate, do you want to go with me and get some steaks?"

"Steaks?" I said. "I love steak (other than gristle)! Sure!"

He said, "Great—get in the truck."

This was awesome. I was going to get to ride with Grandpa in his dump truck. He had his lunch pail and a thermos with coffee, and I felt like a big boy. We went bumping down the road and drove through town right past the *Piggly Wiggly* and I asked him, "Aren't we going to get steaks?"

He said, "They're up here a little bit." So we kept bumping along, and I was thinking, This is a long way; we've been in the truck for over half an hour.

Eventually we stopped at an empty lot with a big muddy hole where several of his guys were standing around. I got out and asked him where the steaks were. He pointed to a bunch of poles poking out of the ground and said, "There you go! There's your stakes! You're here with me all day." It turned out they were building a house, and they'd staked out where they had to sink the rebar. He got his crew going and told me to stay out of the way. I offered to carry their tools so I'd have something to do, but he wouldn't let me. I was stuck there all day long with nothing to do except stare at the sky. He thought that was the funniest story in the world and still tells it sometimes when the family gets together.

Then there was the summer of the puzzle piece when I was eight. It was around a hundred degrees in the trailer, and Blaine and I were sweating over this jigsaw puzzle, around 500 pieces, balloons or mountains; something colorful. At the beginning, I snuck a piece off the table and into my pocket, so when there was only one piece missing I could say, "Hey, look! I've got it!" It was fun for me to put this thing together knowing I had the missing piece and would save the day.

So we finally finished it, but there was one piece missing. We were looking everywhere—under the table and the beds and the rug, and we asked Grandma. She couldn't find it. And then Grandpa got home, and Blaine told him we finished but were missing a piece. Grandpa asked where the piece was. I told him I didn't know, but I was smiling, and then Blaine slowly slunk away into the next room because he knew I was setting myself up for disaster.

Grandpa asked, "Nate, do you have the piece? Now don't lie to me, because you won't like it if I find out you're lying." I said, no, I didn't have it. And he said, "You're lying to me. I'm going to ask you one more time to give the piece up." And I told him again I didn't have it. And he picked me up by the shoulders and started banging me against the wall, which was paneled with wood, and the whole trailer started rocking.

I was crying, but he kept pounding my body against the wall, shouting in my face to give up the piece. I remember crying in pain as I dug it out of my pants pocket. Then he dropped me and said, "Never lie to me again or it will be worse." It was hard to imagine how it could have been worse. My head hurt, my body hurt. I remember the feeling of his huge hands digging into my shoulders, holding my arms really tight. And the sound of it—boom! boom! boom! I remember my grandmother silently leaving the room. My German grandmother, the prototypical movie grandma: short, portly, cuddly (and laughs hysterically). She was always there for a hug, and to laugh with, and play games with, and cook with. She always had snicker doodles that she'd just made or stored in the freezer, and as soon as we got there she'd say, "Let's go and get you cookies!"

I loved my grandmother, but she was afraid of my grandfather and would shut down or disappear at the first sign of his rage. At dinner, if he told me I had to eat something and I said I didn't want it, he'd say to me, "No, you're going to eat it!" I would look at Grandma and she'd be chewing with her head down. When my grandfather was banging me against the wall, she never came to my defense or tried to protect me from his abuse. I still love her. But I think we were both afraid of him.

6

*Don't be afraid
to start all over again.
You may like
your new story better.*

6

In the fifth grade at FIS, 1989, as mentioned before, Tyler was my best friend. He was so cool. He smoked *Lord* cigarettes, so, naturally, I began smoking too. He drank beer, as well. But remember, in Germany beer was legal. They even served kinder beer at school during lunch; beer in little juice boxes with a straw! Yeah, the alcohol content was low, about .05%, but it was beer!

When I was 12 until about 13, Tyler and I would hang out at the cafes and order beer and smoke. My parents had no idea what I was up to. Tom kept working his eighty-hour weeks, and as soon as Mom got home from work she slept most of the day away.

Then there was Blaine; he and I were like cowboys. We'd take the trains everywhere on our own. I'd get home at 2 p.m. from school, and then we'd go out again and not get home until eight or nine at night.

Once I met a guy in his thirties, a janitor in another town, and we hit it off. He took me to his apartment to listen to music. It was the first time I heard Jimi Hendrix. Nothing crazy happened; we just hung out. But my parents never knew about it.

I'd been smoking for at least a year when I finally was caught with my pack of Lords by Tom. I'd spend the time after school at Tyler's house and smoke a few cigarettes so my clothes stank of it. I had been using the excuse that his parents smoked, and I picked up the smell from their house. That worked until Tom caught me going up the hill one day and followed me, wondering what I was up to.

He confronted me as I was lighting up, and I had to admit that it was true. Both Mom and Tom were disappointed but neither exacted any significant punishment on me. I just never smoked at home again.

My mother would occasionally pick me up from school. It was normally a thirty-minute bus ride to and from, but one day she arrived and handed a photo to Blaine and me of a smiley face on a postcard of Jacksonville, Florida. She excitedly told us we were moving back to the US of A! And Florida of all places! I was delighted to leave Germany and everything about it behind.

This was a relief in so many ways. Mom had been very ill, her health had declined terribly, her depression was scary; I was about to be kicked out of school, learning nothing but unacceptable social habits. But that summer of 1991, everything changed.

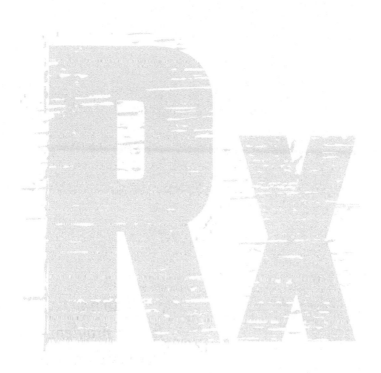

*I do not
fix my problems
I fix my thinking.
The problems
fix themselves.*

—Buddha

7

When we arrived back in the States, my mom became my mom again, at least for a while, until Tom's next nuclear bomb exploded. I was 14 and back in school with kids like me. I immediately had friends; I made the football team; for the first time in years, I felt like I fit in. Tom was making a lot of money, and I was the kid with the big, fancy house beside one of the greens of an exclusive country club, the pool for great parties, and the best cars money could buy—expensive Mercedes and BMWs. I was also the kid whose parents weren't paying close attention to what he was doing, so I could do whatever I wanted. Swimming pools were everywhere and 14-year-old boys with hormones found plenty of interesting girls poolside!

The Orange Park Country Club was a status symbol for Tom. The new home luxurious and, once again, my parents built a pool with all the amenities. The best part of all was that we had a lot of great neighbors with kids who all spoke English. Mom and Tom's room was on one side of the house and mine and Blaine's were on the other, which meant we had plenty of privacy and separation.

In the world at large, the Cold War came to an end (which meant that the pieces of the Wall that Blaine had collected on a previous trip to Berlin were very cool), and I resumed the eighth grade where there was no mention of it, as important as it was. I was too consumed by my entrance to Orange Park Middle School to even care.

Blaine's high school, with older students more aware of world events, was a bit different. In the early 1990's there was racial tension with regard to Rodney King, the LA Riots, and other simmering racial tensions from being in the South in general. I experienced none of that; in fact I became very active in sports for the first time in my life. I loved football, ran track (I was pretty fast), and life was great. My mother was back, and I don't mean just present; she was happy, smiling, swimming, playing on a tennis team, and entertaining Tom's business associates again. Life was amazing— for a couple of years. Then Blaine went off to the University of Florida, and I entered Orange Park High.

We'd been enjoying Jacksonville for a couple of years. Tom had acquired many friends and business associates, so he threw himself a big 40th birthday party at our house. He was on top of the world. There was a full bar set up in the driveway, and when the bartender stepped away, a buddy of mine and I grabbed a bottle of rum and some *Coke* and took it to my room.

I drank a little when we lived in Germany, but I never got drunk. The rum was my first taste of hard liquor, and I loved it. We got shitfaced. It was the best, this burning feeling I got as I drank the rum and Coke. As for taking the bottle, I didn't think of it as stealing; Tom was paying for the bar, so the stuff was ours. If anything, I felt pretty cool, snagging a bottle of rum and no one being the wiser. A part of me knew I shouldn't do it—I was well underage—but that just made it sweeter.

My sophomore year in high school started out with promise, but it went south fast. I was 16, and I got a fake ID so I could buy cigarettes whenever I wanted. I had started smoking all the time. Things between my parents were so tense and estranged that we merely existed in that house; we weren't living. We made it look good, especially when Blaine was home visiting from college. We were the best counterfeit family.

I could smell like pot, cigarette smoke, or alcohol, but my parents never questioned it because they were in their own world, and I was just there. Only I wasn't really there. I was floating in a different world with a new a 5.0 Mustang and a fake ID. I could leave at 11:30 on a weeknight, hang out at a bar, come home at 2 a.m., drag myself to school a few hours later, and no one noticed or said a word. It was as if I didn't exist. I just wanted to feel anything but how I felt when I was at home.

And then there was sex. I wanted to learn about it. One of my buddies had a porn video he passed around, and it was my turn to see it. I'd hidden it in my closet under a stack of dirty laundry because I thought no one would go in there. But I came home one night and found my parents in the living room, waiting up for me. Mom was crying. I thought they were going to tell me that someone had cancer, but no: she had found the video. I was mortified. And then my father gave a big speech about how porn isn't the way women are supposed to be portrayed, that men are supposed to love women and treat them with respect. Looking back on how Tom was treating my mother and his numerous affairs, it's clear that everything he told me that night and throughout my entire childhood was nothing but lies.

I was also starting to experiment with drugs and other stuff. On one occasion, my parents were away somewhere, and I had a bunch of friends over for the weekend. We stayed up all night and at five in the morning, we went out to a cow pasture and picked these hallucinogenic mushrooms—'shrooms, we called them. They grew right out of the cow poop, and they had a little purple ring around the stem so you'd know it was a 'shroom. If you picked the wrong ones, you could die. They grew in Florida because it was so humid at night. They would creep up just as the sun started to rise; they'd last an hour, maybe an hour-and-a-half, then it would get hot and they'd shrivel up and die. The street value was through the roof, but we weren't dealers. We just wanted to have fun.

So we went out and picked a bunch of 'shrooms and brought them back to my house. I got out a big pot, filled it with water, got it boiling, and dumped the 'shrooms in along with the soil, cow poop, the works. We boiled it for about 30 minutes, and the water turned an inky, purple-black color. Then we took a tee shirt and stretched it over a jug, strained the liquid into the jug, and squeezed the 'shrooms in the tee shirt to get the last drop out. We were in the middle of doing this when suddenly I heard the garage door opening, and my friend said, "Uh, I think your parents are here."

They'd come home early—holy shit! I grabbed the pot, set it on a towel in my closet, covered it with dirty laundry (my trusty technique), and ran back into the kitchen just as my parents came strolling in.

I said, "Hi, how's it going? You're home early!" And they said, "Well, you're up early too. Yeah, we decided to come home." And they went to their room. That was it. No questions about the funky smell, or all the stuff on the counter, or what a bunch of teenage boys were doing, fully dressed in the kitchen at 10 a.m. on a Saturday morning. Just, "Hi, guys. 'Bye, guys. See ya."

I began drinking every weekend, sometimes a lot, and also smoking weed and taking the occasional LSD trip. This was when I was driving drunk, scaring my friends, parking sideways in the driveway, and shoplifting. My grades took a nosedive, but I wasn't thinking about what it meant for my future. All I thought about was now I was feeling good. I was having fun. That's all that mattered.

But occasionally did get caught. I remember I fell asleep at a neighbor girl's house and didn't get home until after one in the morning. I was a junior in high school at the time, and my curfew was ten o'clock.

When I walked in, my parents were both sitting there. Tom stood up and slapped me right across the face and told me never to do that again. Yeah, I was late, so ground me, take away privileges. But slap me like that? I was humiliated. And furious. I wanted to hit him back.

But growing up, I really was invisible. If the wildly popular movie Home Alone could have been real, that kid would have been me. No one paid any attention unless I did something wrong. When I racked up speeding tickets and got my license suspended, Tom made it into a father-and-son traffic school adventure. When I told my parents I was getting a five percent in pre algebra, they said, "Do we need to get you tutoring?" I said no, and that was that. I just talked my way out of it.

I snuck out of the house every night and came back smelling of liquor and cigarettes, but they never noticed. They went on vacation for a week when Blaine was at college, so it was just me at the house. I threw an unbelievable party. The next day, a bunch of friends came back and we cleaned everything up. When my parents came home, they said, "Oh, wow, the house looks great. It looks clean!" I said, "We just wanted to make sure everything was nice for you when you got home."

Then my mom walked into our backyard. There was a huge sago cactus right by the pool. She said, "Why are there all these beer bottles and cigarette butts here?" I said, "Well, we had a little get together." And she said, "Oh, you did?" and then she dropped it, no questions asked.

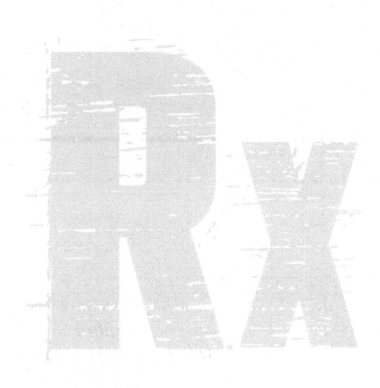

*The present moment
is filled
with joy and happiness.
If you are attentive,
you will see it.*
—Ticht Nacht Han

'd been allowed to run wild as a kid in Germany, and it was the same in Florida. My activity didn't matter. I was always allowed to go out. No one ever stopped me; no one said no. Mom and Tom, if they were around, would say, "Okay, Nate. Be safe or see you later," without even looking up. No boundaries. At the time, it was the best ever. But now that I'm a dad, it's very different. Now I realize I was selfishly and abusively neglected.

For the most part, I was a good kid, but I got cocky and was arrested in 1993 for shoplifting at *Walmart*. They didn't require a receipt to return an item, so I'd steal something expensive that fit in my pocket, take it to a different *Walmart*, and return it for cash. I thought I had the best thing going until my fourth time which ended with me being tackled in the parking lot by a security guard. That got my parents' attention. Tom came down to the police station where he found me handcuffed to a wooden bench. The extent of my punishment from the police was basically a hand slap, and I was grounded by my parents for a couple weeks. I hated that, but deep down, I think it told me there might be a chance they actually cared about what happened to me. They weren't happy I was arrested for shoplifting, but all they did was tell me to get a job after school. The only time I had major consequences was the time I came home stoned and left my car parked across the driveway.

I was going through a psychedelic phase. On Friday nights, my friends and I would drop acid and go out and do silly things. We went to a Mexican restaurant one time and just stared at our plates, laughing hysterically because the rice looked like ants.

Once we dropped acid and went to a horror movie called *Candyman* about a crazed killer who appeared if you stood in the dark in front of a mirror and said his name three times. Afterward, I was in the men's room with a buddy, and I turned off the lights and shouted, "Candyman! Candyman! Candyman!" while he was in a stall, begging me to shut the hell up. I scared that poor guy to death.

Then there was the time I freaked out a friend when I wasn't trying. I was tripping and driving him home after a movie one Saturday afternoon. It was pouring down rain with a lot of traffic, and suddenly my buddy was grabbing the oh-shit handle, his knuckles and face all white. I glanced over and asked him what the problem was, and he screeched that I was driving like a maniac and he was afraid he was going to die. Me? I was having a blast. This was long before I got my first DUI, but I was on my way.

Another time, a bunch of us were on acid and watching The Omen at a friend's house. This guy's parents had religious statues all over the place, which my friend was convinced were possessed and flying around, so I decided to go home, only I couldn't remember how to get there, which was worse than it sounds because I lived a total of three blocks away. I kept driving back to ask directions on how to drive the three hundred yards to my house.

After three hours, I finally made it home, parked in the driveway, and went straight to bed. I was awakened by headlights sweeping my room. My parents had just gotten home. I stayed under the covers pretending I was asleep because it was late, and I was still high and hallucinating that there were spiders on the walls.

Suddenly, my bedroom light was on and my parents were standing there, my mother wailing about me being on drugs and my father growling that I'd better get my ass out of bed and pee in an empty mayonnaise jar. I swore that I wasn't high and didn't know what they were talking about. Then Tom told me to go outside and see how I'd parked the car. I had parked sideways, so the car was straddling the driveway, parallel to the garage door.

"But I got in really late," I said, "and I was super tired." Tom then showed me his watch. It was 8 p.m. That disaster landed me in a Christian high school which my parents thought would whip me into shape. It lasted a week. The experience of the new school was so deeply depressing, my parents finally allowed me to go back to my high school.

I think sometimes that if they had said no to me more often, there would have been a chance I could have learned how to say no to myself. But I never did. Whatever I felt like doing, I did. After that night chugging rum and Coke, I knew I liked the feeling it gave me. I'd hang out at friends' houses and we'd raid their parents' liquor cabinets. We'd still get high on 'shroom juice. I smoked cigarettes and weed, and eventually consumed vast amounts of alcohol. When I was at my worst, I was drinking a handle of vodka every day. That's forty shots. It's amazing I didn't kill myself from alcohol poisoning. I polluted my body with smoke, drugs, and alcohol because I didn't think I mattered.

RX

During high school, I fell head over heels for this girl. We were at a party and started drinking. Before I knew it, we were upstairs on the bathroom floor, in the dark, and I was putting on a condom. I'd had sex once before so I kept one in my wallet because someone told me it was a good idea. And it was, until I turned the lights back on and the girl shrieked that the condom was on the floor and not on me. She straightened her clothes and ran back downstairs, where I found her with a friend, crying like crazy. She said she was sure she was pregnant, and what were we going to do? I was bewildered; how could she know so fast? It had been maybe five minutes. My buddy provided consolation by way of more alcohol. The night was a complete mess.

That was on a Saturday. On Monday, I came home from school and had my usual snack of nachos. I'd crush the Nacho Cheese Doritos in the bag, put them in the bowl with shredded cheese, and microwave them for a minute; then eat it with a spoon! Delicious!

Then the phone rang. It was the girl's brother, and he wanted to know how I was going to pay for this baby. I asked him how he knew she was pregnant and he said, "Oh yeah, she's pregnant all right." He said the test identified me as the father, and if I didn't step up and financially take care of the baby, he and his brother were going to come after me and kick my ass.

You've got to picture the scene: my sorry teenage self, frozen, a phone in my hand, and my Nachos and cheese congealing on the counter. I hung up in a state of panic. I replayed our bathroom encounter over and over in my mind. I knew I'd put on the condom, and it was plenty snug, and we went at it for a little while. She had reached up with her hand and touched me down there, and then it was over. A second later she was crying. What the heck had happened? What went wrong?

These calls went on the rest of the week, now with two of her brothers on the line, threatening me with all kinds of mayhem. I realized I had to get my parents involved, so I sat them down and told them. It didn't go over well. I could see the disappointment in their eyes. But Tom had his head on straight for once, and told me to let him know the next time the goon squad called. They did, later that night. Tom got on the phone. "Look, if your sister is pregnant and you're holding my son responsible, we need to meet at the hospital so she can have a blood test to establish paternity. Call back when you've made the appointment." This was the only time Tom ever stood up for me that I recall.

They never called again. It turned out their sister was indeed pregnant: she gave birth to a full-term baby five months after our encounter. I was stunned. I could not believe that she had conned me like that. She knew I lived in a cool house and drove a hot car, so she figured my family would pay a boatload of money to support the kid. Then it dawned on me that when we were having sex and she touched me, she was actually dislodging the condom. Everything she did that night—the flirting, the sexy talk, the dreamy eyes—was premeditated. She took me for a privileged, horny kid who was too naïve to know you couldn't know you were pregnant in the time it took to walk down a flight of stairs. And she was right. But what she didn't know was that her actions changed how I viewed women for decades. I continued having girl-friends, but it was years before I ever really trusted a woman again. I was extremely careful when it came to sex—no one was going to play me like that again. I didn't take the act or the woman I with seriously; not for a long time.

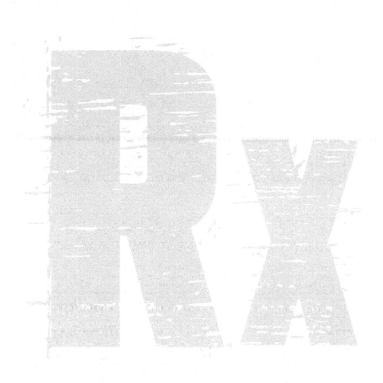

Judge nothing
you will be happy.
Forgive everything
you will be happier.
Love everything
you will be happiest.

—Buddha

9

We'd been in Jacksonville for three years when Mom's cousin Kathy visited us the summer of 1995. She came to spend a couple of weeks and celebrate my mom's birthday; she stayed in our guest room.

We didn't have a lot of family, but Mom was really close to this cousin; they were like sisters. Kathy, a successful dietitian, was four years Mom's senior, living in Missouri, close to our extended family. She had married Scott, a fireman with a great history within his department. We didn't see them often, once or twice a year at best, especially because of our time in Germany. But when we moved to Florida, visits were more frequent and a lot more fun.

It was always a treat with Kathy. We all loved her and she really loved spending time with our family.

I was dating a cute girl, Christine; she was 16 and I was 17 at the time. I was, of course, spoiled rotten by affluent parents living in a very nice neighborhood. All the kids wanted to come and hang out at my house. Shoot, even some of my parents' friends were jealous of me because my folks had gotten me a white 1993 convertible Mustang, a very hot car, and I took Christine everywhere in it.

Driving through the neighborhood one day, I saw Tom's Mercedes up ahead and gunned the 'tang to catch up and say hello. I could tell Mom was in the car with him. Her blond hair was a dead giveaway. But as I pulled alongside, I noticed it was Kathy. For some reason, she was embarrassed and slunk down in her seat. I didn't think anything about it at the time, but she ended up going home a week earlier than expected.

Tom always came home late and Mom, the captain of the Women's Country Club Team, spent her days playing tennis, working out at the gym, shopping, or spending time with her friends. Trying desperately to please her husband, she became severely anorexic. Blaine was off at college. Once again, no one knew where I was or what I was doing. I thought I had it made. What I didn't think about was how it was affecting my schoolwork.

As the end of my senior year neared, I found out my low grade in a pre algebra class would keep me from graduating. The teacher was going to give me a zero but eventually decided to pass me if I spent the last weeks in study hall. So that's what I did. I didn't care; I had no pride. I just listened to music, smoked cigarettes and weed, drank at night, and put on weight. Deep down I knew this wasn't good. It was a tense time. My grandparents had arrived after driving from Nebraska to celebrate my high school graduation. Upon learning I may not graduate, my mom became frantic. I think my parents had given up. Mom was overwhelmed and Tom simply didn't care. Their second son didn't matter. My parents had no idea who I was, really. And the sad fact is that neither did I.

RX

We were all thrilled with the return to our way of life in sunny, beautiful Florida. It was like Johnny Nash's *I Can See Clearly Now* . . .

I can see clearly now the rain is gone
I can see all obstacles in my way
Gone are the dark clouds that had me blind
It's gonna be a bright (bright)
Bright (bright) sunshiny day . . .
Here is that rainbow I've been praying for . . .

But, unfortunately, there was no rainbow for us. The dark clouds had begun years before, began to descend again. They were so intense that I, as a 17-year-old, just wanted to disappear. And alcohol was the only escape I knew.

10

You can't stop the waves,
but you can learn
how to surf.
—Jon Kabat-Zinn

10

om was sitting at the kitchen table, still wearing her bathrobe.

I had just walked in the door from school and she had her head in her hands, sobbing. She didn't look up when I came in nor when I said hello. She just sat staring down at the table. My first thought was that something had happened to Tom or Blaine.

"Mom," I said. No reaction. "Mom? Mom!" She looked up. Her face was stricken and puffy. "Mom, what's up? What's going on?"

"It's your father. He's cheating on me. He wants a divorce."

What? I was stunned. I remember getting tackled in football, hit so hard the wind was knocked out of me, and I didn't know what was happening for a few seconds. This was how I felt when Mom said Tom was cheating.

Tom liked to flirt; we all knew that. I'd seen him in action only a week before at the big surprise birthday party he'd thrown for Mom. He'd always been like that, and she hated it. Why would he spend all that money on a party for her if he didn't love her? Why would he pay for Kathy to come? And the Rolex! Who buys a diamond-encrusted gold Rolex for someone he doesn't love? Mom was emotional, always had been. So I thought she was probably exaggerating.

"Mom, come on. You're probably—"

"Nathan, it's true. He told me about it this morning, right where you're standing. He wants a divorce."

"But who? Who is it?"

"He won't tell me. He just said he's in love with someone else, that he never really loved me in the first place. He wants me to leave."

She looked younger without makeup, like an innocent, broken child. I could see the pain, it was visceral to me. And something came over me. I lost it. I'd heard people talk about seeing red but never understood until that moment, when everything was colored by a bright, red rage. Tom's face floated up in front of me, and I wanted to hit him, hurt him. I didn't care about the consequences.

The next thing I knew, I was in my car speeding downtown. It was a miracle I didn't have an accident because all I remember from the drive was hearing Tom's voice yelling at me the way he always did, about how much I embarrassed him and how decent people don't act like I do; hollering "don't do this" and "don't do that," and all the while he was doing much, much worse.

Then I was pulling up to his office building, still focused on finding Tom. I ran inside. His employees were saying *hi* and *how are you*, but I couldn't respond. I saw him in his glassed-in office. I stormed in, practically shattering the door as I slammed it open and started unloading on him.

He plastered a smile on his face and tried to get around me to close the door, all the while saying with a false underlying chuckle, "Nate, quiet down, now. Ha, ha. Come on, calm down." But when he got close to me, his voice was low and menacing as he growled, "You'd better be quiet. You're in my office. Shut up!" His teeth were bared, displaying an evil grin. I wasn't having any of it.

"I'm not going to be quiet!" I was really shouting now. "How could you do this to Mom? How could you have sex with someone else? How could you break up our family like this? Fuck you, you asshole!"

I spun around and made my way back through the office. Everyone was frozen, staring. I kept moving until I was back in my car headed home. When I looked up, in the rearview mirror I saw a white Mercedes a few cars back. It was him. Thirty seconds later, he pulled into my lane. He was right on my bumper, not more than a dollar bill's length away. If I'd never felt dread before, I felt it now. I knew something bad was going to happen. All the way home, he never passed me, never got alongside me. He just stayed behind, on my tail the entire way.

I swung into the driveway, leapt from the car, and started running to the back of the house. I was prepared for a confrontation but had no idea it would go down the way it did. I heard his car pull in behind me, footsteps rushing up, and then he was on me. We crashed onto the wooden deck. He hit me in the face, hard, and I thought, *Okay, it's on now.* And then, *What am I going to do?*

This was my father beating the shit out of me! He was 42 and I was 17. I was younger, but he had that hardened strength that comes with age and is much more powerful and enduring than that of a kid.

I didn't hit him. But I wanted to kill him. I was ducking, my arms and hands covering my face and wherever else he was hitting me. Cursing and pushing and grunting, we knocked over the deck table. He kept yelling about how I'd embarrassed him at his place of business. That's what he cared about: how he looked to other people. He didn't care that he had broken my mother's heart and destroying our family—no, all he cared about was his magnificent image!

He was still pounding me with his fists, and I was trying to grab his arms to stop him. That's when Mom came running out of the house shouting that she was going to call 911 if we didn't stop. She was standing there with this big, clunky portable phone in her hand, and I thought, I'm done. I am done here. I stood up, backed away from him, and limped off.

I wasn't in any kind of shape to drive, but I had to get away from there. I cried all the way to my friend Danny's house, told him what had happened, that I'd been beaten up by Tom, and I sat there on his bed, sobbing and shaking. He comforted me and told me it would be okay.

"If they get divorced, it's all right," he said. "I've gone through it. You'll be all right." And I thought, *Sure, you're all right, but this isn't you. It's me. This is my family. Was my family.* The world was wondering if Ross and Rachel on *Friends* would ever get back together again. I was wondering about my own parents!

Everything was different now. After a few hours in Danny's room, it began to sink in.

I went home that night after everyone had gone to bed. I didn't want to run into my mom because I couldn't bear to see her pain. And I didn't want to run into Tom because I utterly despised him. That was the beginning of the end of our relationship. I couldn't even call him Dad anymore. He became Tom and has been ever since.

The magnitude of his betrayal and the viciousness of his assault signaled the end of my normal emotional development. Until then I had been drinking with my friends and smoking some weed occasionally. But that experience caused my heart to seize up and it took me seventeen years to find myself again.

When I finally found out that the woman Tom was involved with was Kathy, I was astounded. It abruptly reminded me that Tom had been a pastor, supposedly teaching the word of God to the youth in his parish, as well as neighbors, friends . . . and, ideally, family. Now, it all just seemed surreal. Who was he? If he was capable of having an affair with one of my mother's closest family members, of what else was he capable?

I had been so caught up in my own life, like all kids that age, I thought my parents had a good relationship. Boy, was I wrong. I thought they loved each other. Wrong again. I thought having the coolest house where all the kids wanted to hang out meant I had it made. But I was wrong about that too. It seemed I was wrong about everything. Nothing I believed and thought was solid and reliable.

11

You are the sky.
Everything else
is the weather.

—Pema Chodron

11

When Tom found out he was being considered for the coveted promotion to Vice President, he delayed taking action on the divorce until after my mom could give an Academy Award-winning performance during the interview process held in Dallas, Texas. Little did I know he was also physically abusing her weakened, anorexic body. Back when he beat the crap out of me, everything stopped. I was 17, an adolescent, and I stayed an adolescent until I became sober. I feel as if I've lived three lives: zero to 17 were my childhood years; 17 to 34 were my using years, and 34 to now are my Recovery years.

I distanced myself from my family. Blaine was at college; Mom was frantically trying to please Tom who demanded she never question him or cry in front of him. Overwhelmed and depressed, she began using alcohol and Xanax to survive. Not wanting to see Tom, I snuck out at night and came home at all hours. I was angry, hurt, and lost, and started doing whatever I could to stop feeling that way.

So when something exciting happened, I was all for it.

12

*Self care is
giving the world
the best of you,
instead of
what's left of you.*

—Katie Reed

12

Tom sold the home in Orange Park and in '98; company movers packed and shipped our entire household contents to Arizona. They were expecting me to move with them. We had been staying in a hotel after the house was sold and its contents shipped. On the morning we were to drive our cars to Arizona, we met at *Cracker Barrel* for breakfast. It was then that I told my parents they would be moving without me. I would be staying with my girlfriend and her family. This news shattered my mom, tears dripped down her face and likely onto her pancakes. Tom had no reaction other to dryly remark that all of my belongings would soon be in Arizona.

The relationship with my girlfriend didn't work out, partly because of the realities of living with someone I hadn't known well, and partly because of an incident involving her kid brother and his pot plant; a plant that I agreed to babysit. The pesky plant was discovered by a cop as he walked his dog and spied it through my bathroom window. I spent what little money I had hiring a lawyer who got the charges down from eleven felony counts to one misdemeanor count, My sentence was sixty hours of community service and completing a course on the hazards of drug and alcohol addiction. After I served my sentence, things finally fell apart with her.

I had graduated high school in '96 and was working at an Italian restaurant as a server, but I played golf all day and was a scratch golfer by age 21. I didn't want to serve cannoli forever and knew I needed to decide what to do with my life. Mom and Tom were in Arizona, and although I didn't miss Tom, I did miss my mom. And there are a lot of golf courses in Arizona . . ..

Since I was a pretty decent player, I decided to pursue golf as a career. I enrolled in the Mundus Institute of Golf Course Management, studying the business of how to run a golf course. Mundus was located in Phoenix, off Camelback Road.

My buddy Vince and I drove a *U-Haul* truck and towed my car from Florida to Arizona in five days, all by ourselves, drinking and living the life. It took three of those days just to get through Texas, where we stopped at a gas station whose sign said it was the last stop for a hundred miles. It was dusk and we walked around the outside of the building to use the restroom. When we came out, we were facing a wall that ran the full length of the station, plastered with hundreds of posters of people who were missing. We looked around at where we were, which was just a gas station and nothing else but tumbleweeds, and then we looked at each other and knew that we needed to get out of there or we might end up on that wall.

It was a sobering moment, even though I was far from sober. Looking at those posters, most of them of young people, some of them kids, a sliver of reality pierced the haze. For a moment, I saw my own face on one of those posters. I knew that could be me. It took only a second but I remember it vividly even now, over twenty years later, as a moment of truth.

It took me two years, but I received my Associate Degree in Golf Course Management and golfed well enough to pass the Professional Golfers Association (PGA) Class A status Players Ability Test (PAT). This meant I was now an apprentice-teaching professional. I spent two weeks at their conference in San Diego, after which they set me up with an internship in North Carolina. Mine was to be in Nag's Head where I spent six months. It was fantastic. That's not to say I stayed out of trouble.

13

*This is who I am
and that's good enough.*

13

had graduated Mundus in '99 and was working at Foothills Golf Club when a road rage incident almost cost me my life. I was on the road around 3:30 p.m. for a lesson at 4 p.m. that I was to teach.

As I pulled out of our street onto the main drag, a large truck came right up on my butt. He must have been in a hurry, but I was 20 years old and it infuriated me! You wanna tailgate me, huh? So I decided to make him really crazy. I caught up to an old lady in the next lane who was driving like a snail, then I slowed down and stayed right next to her. There were only two lanes, so he couldn't get around either of us. You want to ride my ass? I thought, Well, you'll ride my ass going thirty-five.

Oh, man—this guy was flailing his arm, blaring his horn, flashing his lights, everything. And I was laughing and laughing. This was hilarious to me. This went on for two or three minutes, and I could see in my rearview mirror that he was livid. Suddenly, the old lady turned onto another street and this guy pulled up on my right, fast, like he was going to sideswipe me. My Mustang rode about six inches off the ground, and he was driving a monster truck that could almost clear my car. He definitely had the upper hand.

I saw the light turn red and I thought, Oh, shit! I could not be at a red light next to this guy because I'd just pissed him off for five minutes. So now I was pumped up with fear.

He was more than angry. So I said screw this and went right through the red light—and he did the same thing. Now I knew he definitely wanted to inflict some sort of pain on me.

I was now going about eighty in a thirty-five mile an hour zone, and all I could think of was *Back to the Future.* Remember the DeLorean? Right then I wished I'd had that stainless steel car which would have afforded a little more protection. And, then I started to laugh because I also remembered that all DeLoreans have speedometers that only go to 95, and I was about to reach jump speed, 88 mph, at any second!

I was thinking, I hope I get pulled over because he can't kill me if a cop's right there. But of course, no cops were around. So I flew around the corner and into the entrance to the golf club. There's a place in front where you pull up—the bag drop. I was hauling ass and went straight into the bag drop. There was a bunch of people standing there at the time. Fortunately, the monster truck didn't turn in. He just kept going straight. I got out of the car and everyone was concerned for me. "Dude, you're sweating—what's going on?" I mean, I almost keeled over, my heart was pounding so hard. I just said I had been running and was still cooling down. *Yeah, right.*

I could have gotten myself killed that day and I knew it, but somehow I got through the lesson I had to teach and had some drinks to calm down. That's how it was back then. Something terrifying like that drive to the golf course, drinks to calm me down, then pretending to be happy, and do my job like nothing had happened.

But did this experience teach me anything? Hell, no. In fact, my drinking took a major upward swing at this point.

My buddy Casey, who also worked at the Pro Shop, and I

got together one night at his place with few other friends and started drinking. After about an hour of boozing, Casey and I got in his Camaro, and we and our friends went to a local bar about ten minutes away in Phoenix.

There we drank, drank, and drank . . . having a good 'ole time until about 11 p.m. That's when my good friend Ace came over to me to tell me that Casey had urinated all over the floor up at the bar, and the bartender was threatening to call the cops if we didn't get him out of there.

Casey was obviously seriously drunk at this point. We quickly paid the bar tab. I was tasked to drive Casey's Camaro back to his home with him in the passenger seat. Ace was in his car in front of me to make sure we made it back to Casey's apartment.

We were waiting at a street light turning left when the light turned green. I was so drunk, I started honking my horn like a jackass at Ace to go. Just my luck, there was a Phoenix deputy on his motorcycle at the gas station right across the street who heard me doing this. When I made the turn, he quickly pulled up behind me. He could see I was driving erratically.

I turned into Casey's apartment complex and pulled up to enter the gate code. I thought I was home free until the cop pulled his motorcycle right up to me and shouted for me stop and not drive through the gate. It scared me because I didn't even know I was being followed by a policeman.

I stopped and saw Ace drive off as he saw the situation with the cop pulling me over. I don't blame him. The cop then asked me if I had been drinking. At this point, I just went on autopilot and said yes. He had me turn off the car.

Before I could get out, Casey started yelling at him saying that I was driving him home, and we were there and to leave us alone. The cop then went around to the passenger side and pulled him out. Before I knew it, Casey threw a haymaker punch at him.

All of this happened as backup cops arrived on the scene. I watched Casey get tackled by five cops all at once. It was truly like a scene out of a movie. After a few minutes wrestling him down and handcuffing him, the original cop came back over to me and asked if I would take a breathalyzer test at a substation across the street.

I had no idea what my rights were or what I was supposed to do, so I just went along with him like a little scared sheep. I took the breathalyzer test and failed it by being over twice the legal limit to drive in Arizona. He arrested me, but what came next was a surprise. He said he could take me to jail like Casey, or he could take me home; but I had to show up for a mandatory court appearance in the next few days. I opted to go home.

Unfortunately for me, my car and keys were at Casey's apartment. I ended up in front of my parents' house where I lived at the time. It was 3 a.m., and I had to ring the doorbell. I woke Mom and Tom. They came to the door after a few minutes, saw me drunk, and the cop leaving. They asked what happened. I told them I was arrested for DUI. This was the worst feeling in the world: to see mom's disappointment, Tom's irritation, and experience the shame and guilt. It was almost too much to bear.

I went to my room and stared at the ceiling, trying to go to sleep, but replaying the whole disaster in my head. The next day I found out Casey was in jail and charged with felony assault of a police officer.

I retrieved my car when I sobered up and eventually went in to be processed at the jail where I was incarcerated for five days and had my license suspended for a year. I made the decision to immerse myself in work and try to stay out of trouble.

14

*There is no traffic
on the extra mile.*

14

fter taking a couple of weeks to visit my buddies in Florida, I returned to Arizona to my parents' house and rang the bell, but no one answered. It was nighttime and the house was dark, so I got out my key, but it didn't work. I walked around to the back door, but that was locked as well, and, once again, my key didn't work.

I called Mom and told her I was locked out and asked when she'd be back. She said, "Oh, I'm sorry; unbeknownst to me, Tom listed the house while I was visiting my parents in Nebraska."

I stood on the doorstep amazed while she told me she was finally divorcing Tom. He kept the money from the sale of the home and had already moved to Seattle. She had moved to an apartment nearby and invited me to stay. The house sold rapidly and they needed to move things out quickly, so they had a huge garage sale. She also mentioned a lot of my things were sold too. What they hadn't sold was at my mom's apartment, and she said that, of course, I was welcome to come and pick it up.

This had happened in the two weeks I was gone to Florida. I was devastated, standing there like a beggar outside my own home. But it turned out I didn't live anywhere, and my family was gone. I was literally homeless.

But, here I was in my early twenties, and I had a great job teaching golf. Right? Finally, things began looking up in my life.

I met a nice girl, Amanda. She was terrific—super nice, gorgeous, very positive, and agreeable. We became serious pretty quickly. She even moved to Scottsdale when I relocated there.

But for some reason, I began to find fault with her. I'd ask her where she wanted to have dinner or which movie she wanted to see. She'd always let me choose anyway, saying she didn't really care where we ate or what we saw because she just enjoyed being with me. Now that I'm sober, I realize what a gift that was—a woman who liked me as I was and wanted to be close—but at the time, I told myself she just wasn't challenging enough. So I broke up with her and shattered her heart.

After that, I dated plenty of challenging women and wondered what the hell I'd been thinking. I wasn't thinking. I was feeling anxious because this amazing woman had wanted to get close to me, and I was afraid she wouldn't like what she saw when she got to know me more deeply. Instead of facing the feeling and telling her the truth, I deliberately destroyed the relationship. Talk about self-destruct!

My work at the Foothills Golf Club paid me 70 percent commission on all the lessons I taught. It was a sweet deal. There was no end to the number of people wanting lessons and with a high commission, I was making enough money to support my then lifestyle. Plus I spent six months learning from real golf course pros how to handle the business end of golf.

A disappointing turn of events occurred when Foothills decided to sell to another golf course group. Since Foothills was privately-owned, and I only made a commission on my lessons, when they were bought out by this new company, my commission dropped to 30 percent. This meant I could no longer afford to work there. I had to find another job.

15

Let go,
let God.
—AA

15

When I left Foothills in 2001, I found a job with TekSystems, an IT recruiting company in Phoenix. I had no background in that kind of work, but I had made a lot of friends at Foothills, people with some stature in local business. One man in particular liked me and hired me solely because he felt I had great interpersonal skills and his company needed people who could be personable and communicate. He thought that was me, so he offered me a position.

Going from a great job outdoors that I loved to working inside an office building sixty hours a week was a disaster. I hated it. I lasted a year or so. Because I was miserable, my quality of life went straight downhill.

One weekend, I decided to go to Las Vegas with some of the guys from the office. I was making thirty grand a year after paying bills and having some fun, so I managed to save $1600.

Between cocktails on the plane and at the hotel, I was already pretty drunk by the time we got to Vegas Friday night. When we got to the casino, the guys told me to set a limit, so I decided on $200 for the weekend.

My first bet was fifty bucks on roulette, which I lost. (Never play roulette . . . you will always lose.) My second bet was a hundred bucks; I lost that too. I was down a hundred and fifty bucks after about a minute. I was shocked—I didn't realize you could lose so much so fast—but I put on a phony persona and acted like it was fine.

I went to the cage to get more cash, gave them my bank information, and withdrew $600 from my savings account; the casino skimmed a 10% commission. I had $540 dollars in my pocket. I was flush with cash, all of which had come out of my savings, but, whatever. I felt like I was going to be a winner!

I put down three hundred bucks on roulette and lost it—a punch in the gut. Now I was down $450 in three spins. I felt like a zombie. I walked around copping free drinks and looking for a lucky table to join. I won a little at blackjack; now my pocket had $300 in it. I went back to roulette, bet it all, and lost. I had blown $750 in one hour. I was in shock. I ran into my coworkers but acted upbeat. "Hey, let's have dinner! Let's get some drinks!" No one knew.

I went back to the cage after dinner. I had about a thousand dollars left in my account, and I asked the gate lady to withdraw all of it. She looked at me—I remember this—and she said, "Are you sure?" I told her, of course I was sure. She kept $100 commission, handed me $900, and off I went.

I lost it all. Lost every single penny the first night I was there, thinking, I'm cursed! God's against me! I had to go home Sunday and ask my mom for a loan. I was too ashamed to tell her why and made up a story about money being tight and all. I paid her back over time.

That's the sickness I have. I knew it was a bad idea, but I did it anyway. I told myself, This is so bad, it's good. That was the sickness talking; that's what I told myself: *Nate, you're going so far beyond your limits, it's scary good. This is so scary, fuck it—I'm going.*

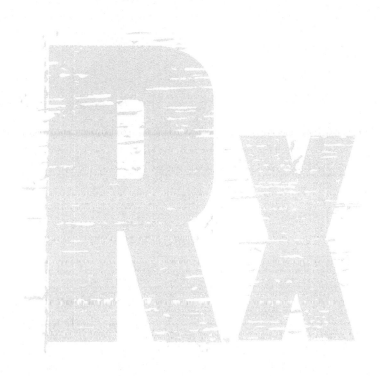

16

*Worry ends
when faith begins.*

16

Once Tom left, Mom found professional help and started her own recovery journey. She also went back to school. She jokingly says now that she studied psychology because she didn't think she could afford all of the counseling she was going to need.

Enrolled full time at Ottawa University, she was working every weekend and finally finding the courage to divorce Tom. Discovery made by her divorce attorney revealed that, over the course of years, Tom had been secretly liquidating their investments by forging her signature. He had also fraudulently canceled and liquidated her life insurance. Even though Tom had made millions during his career, after her twenty-seven year marriage she was left with hardly any money. Tom was gone, all their assets were gone, but she remained.

Eventually, Mom realized her goal and graduated with a Master's degree in Professional Counseling and a second Master's in Traumatic Abuse. Her internship was completed at a treatment center in Wickenburg, Arizona, and when they offered her a full-time position, she stayed.

I was living in an apartment in Scottsdale, so I'd drive up to see her once every couple of months. She was earning enough to buy a nice little house on the desert mesa. I helped her maintain it when I visited so she could plant things. It was nice to still have her in my life.

I visited around her birthday at the end of May. Tom was now back in Phoenix, still working in the same field. Out of the blue, one day he called to ask if I would do him a favor. He said he had something to give Mom, and he felt that what he was giving her would make things right. He said it might get them back together, but he wanted to keep it a surprise.

I was shocked since I seldom, which was pretty much never, heard from him. It had been about six years since our fight in Florida. Things really changed after that. Not only had I stopped referring to or calling him Dad because of how he destroyed our family, but because of how he acted when my friends were around.

There was time back when we lived in Florida where I had friends over, male and female, and we were in the kitchen getting snacks and drinks to bring on our way out to the pool in the backyard. And here comes Tom, completely naked, walking to the hot tub, in front of all of us. Everyone was freaking out. I'm sure they were thinking, "Oh, my god!" And he just says, "Oh, hi!" So we stayed inside. I realized then I could never think of him as "Dad" again. He was no dad; he was no father to me. I had to acknowledge his existence, but I did not have to call him dad. So I called him Tom. I was good with that.

Back to the favor . . .. Even though Tom had had multiple sex partners, various girlfriends, and wreaked havoc on my mom to the point of divorce, I thought he was still trying to work things out with her, and the possibility of our family getting back together was something I dreamed of. There was real hope (one of the best four-letter words ever). I was excited. Here I had the chance of being a part of bringing a little joy, so I hoped, to my mom. I drove to Tom's place, and he gave me a big, flat package; so big it took up my entire back seat.

I drove to Mom's place in Wickenburg, and she opened the door. I was standing there with this box. I told her it was a surprise from Tom, it was from his heart, and he said he hoped she'd love it.

She asked me to carry it into her room, which I did, and then I went back to the kitchen to grab a snack. The next thing I knew, I heard her scream. I went running to the bedroom, but she wouldn't let me in. She finally came out and shut the door behind her and said she didn't want me to see what I'd brought home because, in her words, it was not a nice gift. She was horrified. I learned later it was a poster-sized photo of Tom's erect penis. He'd had it custom-framed.

Mounted underneath the photo was their wedding ring which he'd had cut and flattened so you could read my mother's initial inscription, something like *Forever Yours*. Underneath the ring, he'd written, *Fuck You*. Mom told me this. She would never let me see it. I called him to ask him what the hell, and all he did was laugh his maniacal laugh, like Jabba the Hutt, the alien gangster from *Star Wars*, only a couple of octaves higher. He was nuts, and still is. That's all there is to it.

I remember driving back home thinking, *What the hell just happened?* I was so confused, furious, and, strangely terribly sad, not just because of the obscene 'gift,' but because even the idea that my parents might get back together was hopeless—and I'd played a role in it. Why did someone I wanted so badly to be able to trust lie to me and use me in such a heinous way? He conned me into to hurting and humiliating my mother. Ever since then I keep thinking, *Really? I was a part of this?* These same kinds of things happened again and again; whenever I had contact with him, it was always a recipe for disaster. I wanted to distance myself from him as far as I could, but I soon discovered that was going to be impossible, at least for a time.

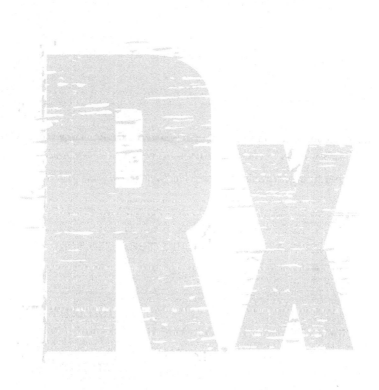

17

You only fail when you stop trying.

17

Even though I was good at it, TekSystems wasn't for me, so while I was trying to decide where to go from there, Blaine suggested I join Tom's new insurance agency in Jacksonville. I wasn't sure I wanted to do that, but I knew I wanted to go home. The straw that "broke" my camel's back was when Tom literally called and begged me to join him. Blaine and I would handle home and auto, and Tom would handle investments and life insurance. I didn't have anything else in terms of offers, so I considered it and decided to give it a chance. Stupidly, I still wanted so much to have a normal relationship with Tom.

So he prepared to fly out to Arizona and help me drive all my stuff back to Jacksonville. While I waited for his arrival in a few weeks, I had some free time on my hands while I packed up and got ready for the trip.

My friends ended up throwing me a farewell party of sorts. My buddy Jason and a few other friends and I went to our favorite bar. They wanted to say goodbye over a night of drinking. We overdid it, as usual, and ended up heading to another bar in Scottsdale, not too far from where I was living. Around 2 a.m., we were hugging and saying goodbye. I will always remember Jason looking at me and asking if I was alright to drive home. He said he'd call me a cab, but I declined and assured him I was good to drive. He knew better, I knew better, but doing the right thing while intoxicated is so fucking hard to do.

Anyway, we all got in our respective vehicles, and I started driving home. A night out drinking always made me hungry, so I stopped at a local grocery store and picked up a frozen pizza and some extra Parmesan cheese to go along with it. I could only imagine how drunk I looked to the cashier at that time in the morning. I got back in my car and rolled the windows down and headed to my apartment.

I was listening to *OutKast* in the car, the sound blaring, but the speed limit was something of which I was very aware. I did not want another DUI. But that didn't stop a cop who had his lights off and was waiting for me down a side street. He pulled out, his lights still off, and tailed me until I failed to use my signal when I was turning into my apartment complex. Imagine the odds of almost getting home for both of my DUIs?

> *You think you've got it*
> *Oh, you think you've got it*
> *But got it just don't get it when there's nothin' at all*
> *—OutKast*

He turned his lights on and pulled me over right at the front of my complex. I couldn't believe it. I thought I was home free.

But no; here was another cop coming to my window while I was shit-faced. He asked all his cop questions, smelling the booze on my breath as I lied about not drinking. It wasn't hard for him to arrest me and take me to the county jail. There I refused the breathalyzer, thinking that was my saving grace; but no, he got some piece of paper from a judge late at night to get a sample of my blood.

I sat in the county jail with cops surrounding me, telling me that I could either abide by the law and have them draw my blood, or they would all hold me down and take it. I was fucked and felt that I just screwed my life up again. In that very second in time, it fractured me.

The jail nurse took my blood; I was put in a cell where I spent the night with other drunks; other arrested individuals came and went out of this cell where I just laid on the concrete cot and thought of all the shit that had come my way.

The next morning, they released me, gave me my arrest papers, and ordered me to appear at my next court hearing. But this time, it was my second 'extreme' DUI which meant I was going to jail for between 60 and 120 days, so I was told.

I walked home, about thirty minutes from the county jail, to my apartment complex. I got to my car and saw a note on the windshield. Someone had hit my car and caused a nice dent but nicely left their contact info. I never called. I just went home and laid in bed, pondering how I was almost home again and messed up so badly.

I felt not just unlucky, but damned. God was out to get me for all the other nights I drove drunk. At that point I made a decision. Run. I was leaving for Florida in the next few weeks. No one knew I had been arrested, so I thought, Hey, fuck it; just go to Florida. After a few years this will all go away. Boy was I wrong, but it felt like the right thing to do. So I didn't show for my court appearance. The city of Scottsdale issued an arrest warrant for me that followed me for the next sixteen years. It took me that long to finally decide to face it.

*Work it
because you are worth it.*
—AA

18

After Tom drove me and my stuff back to Florida, he offered me a glorious future, another lie I chose to believe. Why would I trust him? But I was a 24-year-old child, wanting desperately to be able to trust him, to know he loved me, and wanted what was best for me; I would have done anything to have that become a reality.

I hardly had any money left after that Vegas weekend, but I did have $8000 from an account my parents had opened for me when I was a kid. That's another thing—the account had around $150,000 in it until my parents split up. Tom withdrew almost all the money—his name was on the account—and left me with $8000. I was royally pissed off, but the story I told myself was that he was Tom; he was the one who had given me the money, so, strictly speaking, it was as much his as it was mine. Besides, he must have needed it. And he'd promised I'd make a lot of money working with him and Blaine, so everything was good. Right?

It wasn't, of course. I wanted to trust him so badly, I pretended he was someone he wasn't, and I became someone I wasn't. Part of me saw what was happening, but I didn't want to see it. I pretended to be blind, which was funny, because remember when I was little, they used to call me "the finder." When someone lost something, I was always able to find it. My mom lost a diamond bracelet once and couldn't find it anywhere. I went looking and found it out in the grass in the backyard. She couldn't believe it. (I still love finding things, which is why I run a thrifting business today.) But when I went back to Florida, I couldn't see a thing. Wouldn't see a thing.

Tom's agency was doing well but it was strange working with him. Not only that, for a while we both lived with Blaine's family in their apartment in Jacksonville; their living room was my bedroom. Tom had nowhere to go when he returned from Washington, so it reminded me of the 70s TV show, *The Odd Couple*. Boy, were we the odd couple, but not in a funny way.

When Blaine and Suzanne bought a house, I was no longer living on the floor and finally had a bedroom. It was an improvement, but still, there's not much you can do with a salary of a hundred bucks a week. Tom, at this time, married a client of his whose husband had died, so he moved in with her. His goal was to get her insurance money but she was savvy enough to prevent that and promptly divorced him.

Every once in a while, Tom would do something nice, like when he offered to take my Mustang down to the DMV and get new Florida tags because I couldn't afford it. That was very decent of him, and it was great to be able to drive my car again—that is, when I could afford to buy gas.

When I moved back to Florida, I decided to ignore the reality of my two DUIs. I ushered in an era of personal anxiety that haunted me for years. It was like living with one eye always on my rearview mirror, watching for the cop who I was sure would pull me over one day, find out about the warrant, and throw me in jail. My career was stymied: I had an insurance license, but I couldn't apply for either a current Florida driver's license or a mortgage broker's license because the background check would have turned up the warrant. I became too anxious to drive on the highway or over bridges; I lived in a quiet state of panic that I could relieve only by drinking more and more and more. And the more I drank, the more tenuous my grip on reality became.

After a year or so, things at work weren't going that well. The agency was losing money, which was strange. We had a beautiful office with new, and may I say, expensive furniture, and I was bringing in a lot of business, so I thought everything was fine. But in the two years I worked there, every couple of months, we laid off a staff member, one by one, until it was just the three of us.

I was stunned one morning when a man in a suit swept in with an armed security guard, planted himself in front of the door, and announced, "Everybody, step away. Don't touch anything. You're fired. Get out." Just like that.

We watched while they carried out the computers, the files, and the phones. They let us back in, but we were out of business; the home office shut us down. I knew that Tom had been mouthing off to the managers and some corners were being cut, but I never thought it would come to this.

We eventually were forced to sell the agency for ten cents on the dollar. Chuck Johnson was the buyer and he offered me a job because I knew all the clients. I accepted and got an apartment near the office. There was a college nearby, so I started partying with students at my place. I was 26 and drinking every weekend, plus one or two days during the week. I wasn't a full-blown alcoholic yet, but not far from it.

Besides, Tom was still there and always seemed to keep life interesting.

I had a girlfriend at the time. We had a big party at Blaine's one night and she came. But after she got home, she called to tell me that Tom had scared her. He had cornered her and asked how she and I were doing. She told him we were doing fine, but he kept questioning her about our relationship, and then he said he wanted to date her when we broke up!

As if that wasn't creepy enough, he asked her if she was enjoying the sex she and I were having. She got up to leave then—she'd heard enough—and Tom laughed and said, "I already know about how good the sex is. I taught Nate everything he knows." Can you imagine a father coming on like that to his son's girlfriend and saying such things?

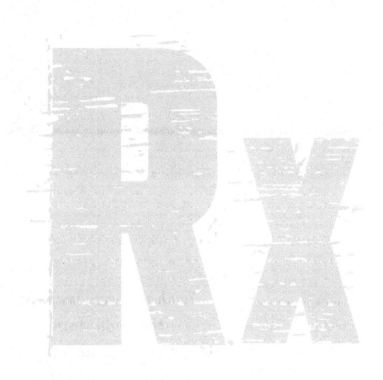

19

*You have been assigned
this mountain
to show others
it can be moved.*

19

Now, with my own apartment, supplied with the bare essentials, I had a home. I would buy multiple half gallon bottles of Smirnoff at the liquor store down the road; and don't forget about my pack a day smoking habit. Drinking and smoking were fused together like peanut butter and jelly. They were the perfect pair. My deck overlooked a parking lot, so I just drank and smoked Kool 100's every chance I got.

Mom was living in Arizona after her graduation from Ottawa in the fall of 2004 and received an excellent job offer from Pine Grove Behavioral Health and Addiction Services in Hattiesburg, Mississippi to start their women's center. This was an incredible opportunity, so she headed to the deep South.

I was very good at selling insurance and helped my new boss to gain some high awards with the company. So I'd sell insurance by day and drink and smoke by night. This went on for nearly a year until I moved into a house Tom bought off Chambore Drive in Jacksonville.

He convinced me to build my credit by entering into a rent-to-lease option with him. Since I'd always paid cash for anything up to this point in my life, I had no credit history at all. I didn't need one since I wasn't planning on buying anything. I had a car that was paid for, I had no intention of buying a home—it was a no-brainer for me.

Tom said I needed a high credit score if I ever wanted to buy a house, so I listened to him as he led me down the garden path again, counseling me to collect as many credit cards as I could, buying furniture on credit, and then holding balances on the cards; all of which is the worst advice someone could ever give to one who never had credit.

So suddenly I had four credit cards totaling 10K and bought 5K in furniture. Mind you, I still only made about $30K from work. Needless to say, I just went crazy buying stuff and maxed out the cards and was now stuck with a ridiculous credit balance at the end of each month. Soon, I couldn't afford the minimum monthly payments.

Once again, I just said *fuck it* and stopped paying on them. Instead of building credit, I wrecked my credit in under a year. I was stuck at Tom's rental with high rent and a credit score that would prevent me from ever actually being able to buy the house. It was a terrible situation, but I always had enough money to stuff the freezer full of vodka and drink my problems away.

Rx

My life was a bore. I lived alone, had no steady girlfriend, and just worked (which I hated) and drank. I dabbled in the occasional cocaine binge with my buddy Robert. He had a hook up with a girl who would always get some coke if he asked.

On a Friday night, he came over to my house, and we began drinking. It was a long work week for me, and I wanted to cut loose. He called his girl and she dropped off an eight-ball of coke. He and I dove into it and then went out to a bar downtown. We partied all night. When we got home, we weren't

NATHAN KRUSE   101

tired, so we partied till the sun came up. Saturday morning rolled around, and I was already drinking vodka and doing coke from the night before. It just continued into Saturday and into Saturday night. No food, just drinking and doing coke.

Sunday morning came, about 8 a.m., and my kitchen was full of empty bottles of booze, beer, and an empty pizza box. We were in the guest bathroom at my house snorting the last of the coke through a $5 dollar bill. I looked at my friend and blood was coming out of his nose and onto the bill. He passed it to me, and I thought nothing of it. I just shoved it up my nose and finished off the drugs. He drove home after that.

I was by myself, starting to come down from all the shit I had just done. I had a ton of work I needed to do in less than 12 hours. I was so depressed and down at this point that I just didn't want to go on with life. I didn't want to kill myself; I was just so sad that I was alone and felt like shit that I didn't want to do anything. Regardless, I got up the next morning with a massive hangover and cocaine still running through my veins and went to work.

I always showed up no matter how hungover I was. I always produced for my bosses no matter how jaded and pissed off I was to work for them. I was paid crap but produced like gold. They only threw me enough scraps to keep me coming back. I needed the booze and the money for rent.

This period of time in my life was horrible. I tried my best to be a good person, but I hated and loathed everything I was. I had a suspended driver's license, I had no money, and a terrible credit score. I was just existing and not living. These were truly the lost years of my life.

RX

I have had a degenerative condition of the spine most of my life, so in January of 2007, Mom picked me up at a hospital in Jacksonville after a nasty surgery. It hadn't gone well. The pain was horrible. I hadn't had a drink since before the surgery so I was feeling pain on a number of levels and wanted someone who wasn't my mom to understand what I was going through and maybe come over later, maybe with a bottle.

So I called one of my good friends and he said he was on his way to a bar to meet some guys and didn't want to talk. It didn't even register with him that I'd just checked out of the hospital and *needed* him.

It had been two months since I'd quit smoking after my surgery. But at home the next day, I decided to have a pity party. I found myself sitting in a chair in the garage, staring at my golf bag, which I hadn't been near in months, and wondering if there were any cigarettes in it. I dragged myself over to the bag and started opening all the zippers until I found a crushed pack. There was one still intact, but it was old.

I limped into the house, turned the stove to high—it was electric, smooth-top—and when it was glowing all orange, I lit the cigarette. It tasted so stale, but I didn't care because it gave me such a head rush. I got high for a second. It had been months since I'd smoked and I was like, *Wow!* I sat back down in the garage, smoking that old cigarette because it was so delicious! And it was taking away all my thoughts of angst, depression, and being pissed off. The taste, the nicotine, all of it. It blew my mind how good it made my body feel. It made my head fuzzy, it relaxed me. I smoked it down to the filter and said, 'F' this, drove to gas station, and got two packs of Kool 100s. I kept smoking for five more years.

RX

Then in April of 2007, I met the love of my life. Lizzy was jogging through my neighborhood, training for a half marathon. I was parking my car after a long day at the office, smoking a cigarette, which I never did as I would always go into the backyard to smoke. But there I was smoking, and I see this hot looking young thing come running past me. The Chambore house was located in a small neighborhood, so I knew she wasn't living there. I saw her run by and she smiled at me. I smiled back and then she was gone. I went inside, thinking nothing of it, and poured myself a drink.

The next day after work I was sitting on my porch, and I looked up. Here she came again, running, but this time she had a dog with her. It was raining a little, and she ran by me, and we again exchanged smiles. I thought to myself, *Wow! This is fate to see this mysterious woman two times in two days.*

I called my best friend Vince and told him about her and swore that if I saw her again I would ask her out. So later that week, Friday night, I was setting up for a neighborhood garage sale with my brother and his family for Saturday morning. We were out there drinking and having fun putting all our stuff out to sell on tables when my buddy told me to look down the street. I did and I saw *her* coming my way. I worked up the courage and stopped her as she was walking by with her dog again. I asked her if she would like to come by our garage sale the next morning. So dorky, but she said she might. I was over the moon. Saturday came and I was out there, hungover, but had my trusty cup of vodka and soda water when Lizzy showed up with a friend in tow.

I jumped over my niece sitting on the curb and introduced myself again. I pulled Lizzy away from the crowd and told her probably the worst thing you could say to a stranger. I said, "Hey, I've seen you running a few times, and I think it's fate that you showed up this morning. Here's my business card. Call me if you'd like to get together one day." Believe it or not, she called me Monday morning and our romance began.

Rx

I was in love, but my romance with Lizzy had some major ups and downs. I'd fallen head over heels for her. I wanted to start a family. I was 30 and she was 25 at the time, having just received her CPA license with the whole world in front of her. After a few more rocky months together, she made the choice to move to NYC. I was completely devastated. But how could I blame her? I was an absolute drunk, hitting my prime of alcoholism.

I was crushed when she left at the beginning of 2008. My life went into a tailspin of negativity. It was really hard to keep going. This time I relied on the vodka more than ever to fill the void in my broken heart. Lizzy and I stayed in touch, but I was infuriated with myself and the fact I had abused drugs and alcohol for so long. I was falling apart and, at this point in my life, I cast God out.

Rx

It was summer of 2008, and I was drinking heavily, trying to close the wound in my heart after Lizzy left for New York. I came home one day and to my surprise I saw a big white and orange cat sitting by my front door. I had lived there at the house for three years now and never once saw a cat. Well, I didn't do anything other than walk by it and go inside for the night.

The next day, there was the cat again, and I started thinking, *Should I feed this thing? Give it water?* I asked my neighbors if they knew this cat and they didn't but did say if you feed it, it will never leave you. So I didn't feed the cat as I didn't want a pet or the responsibility of anything other than keeping my vodka cold in my freezer.

The third day rolled around, and as I pulled in to the driveway there was this cat again. I went inside, ignoring it, and made a drink. I was sitting on the back porch, bored, and all of a sudden this cat jumps out of nowhere and starts meowing and rubbing against my leg so sweetly. I asked my neighbors for some dog food as that's all they had. I opened up the can and gave it to the cat and watched it devour that food like no one's business.

My neighbor watched as the cat ate the dog food and asked me, "Now that you've fed it, what are you going to call it?" I wasn't sure, but she said it's crazy that a cat just appeared out of nowhere and here he is at your house to be your friend— and that was that; his name was going to be Justappear, and we became fast friends.

I wouldn't let him stay inside my house and only fed him once a day outside. But after a few weeks of him loving on me and always being there when I got home, I decided to allow him in. That was the trend with Justappear. I would say I wouldn't let him get too close, like letting him in my room or on my bed, but after a while, he was snuggled at my feet as we fell asleep.

I believe now, looking back, that Justappear was sent to

me to keep me alive until I got sober. With his unwavering love and always waiting for me, it gave me a reason to be home at night. It gave me a reason to wake up and feed him. I enjoyed having him around as I could tell he appreciated my company. He was grateful I fed him good food and petted him whenever he wanted. It was like two lost souls finding each other at the right time. We formed a special bond over the years, and he eventually moved with me four times while I was drinking myself to death.

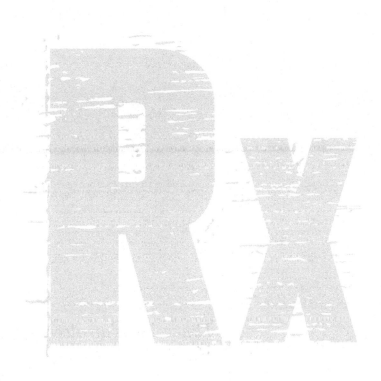

20

*I knew I was an alcoholic
by the way I felt sober.*

—John B., AA

20

In 2009, when I left the Chambore house and moved to an apartment in Orange Park, I lost all contact with Tom. I heard bits and pieces about him through Blaine, but that was about it. Tom came to pay me a visit one time at 5 a.m., banging on my front door asking for money. I told him I barely had any money myself; but he was so desperate for $100. He wanted to take some woman and her child to the zoo for the day. I gave it to him so he would leave.

It was weird seeing him like that; desperate and broke but still trying to impress a woman. I had so much anger toward him at this time from all the years—literally decades of abuse and lies.

My friend Vince and I were drinking and happened to be driving by Tom's house one day, and I decided to go see what that asshole was up to. Mind you, I was drunk and full of anger so this wasn't going to go well.

He was home and saw us drive by, so I stopped and got out to confront him. Things got heated quickly, and I pushed him down and started hitting him. Vince got in the way, broke it up, and I went back to my Jeep and started to hit my steering wheel with my fist. I was seeing red and Vince asked what the hell was going on? I took off and never looked back.

I didn't know or care what Tom was doing and wasn't going to waste a moment's thought on him ever again. It wasn't until 2011 when Blaine told me the FBI had arrested Tom for executing a Ponzi scheme and ripping off multiple families. While his trial was in progress, he compounded his problems by attempting to hire a hit man to kill two key witnesses who happened to be undercover FBI Agents, so he got a few more decades added to his sentence.

Tom is currently incarcerated in a Federal prison somewhere in the US. Hopefully, he will serve his full sentence and not have an opportunity to inflict his pain on anyone else for a long, long time. I believe we each have our feet firmly planted exactly where they are at and his happen to be in a 6 by 8 concrete cell for thirty years.

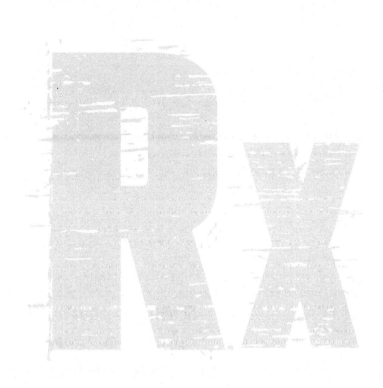

21

> "Serenity is what we get
> when we quit hoping
> for a better past.
>
> —NA

21

With God eliminated from my life, I committed myself to worshiping at the altar of a new Holy Spirit—the spirit of *Smirnoff* vodka.

My life had now come full circle. I was back in my old neighborhood complete with bad memories. I worked and drank heavily, so much now that when I woke up my eyes were puffy like an old man's. They were so swollen that the people I worked with asked if I'd had a fight and gotten punched.

I drank and drove so much that my anxiety was accelerating. I'd already had a problem with driving over bridges, but I began experiencing this phenomenon even more. Jacksonville is known for its many bridges, so it was hard to not drive over them. I would get the feeling that I was going to pass out and drive right off the side of one. My hands would get slippery with sweat and my heart would pound. It was so bad that if I knew I had to drive over a bridge, it would consume my thoughts.

I drove with a bottle of vodka in my car then, and I always had a drink in my hand. *Always.* I was in a continuous state of drunkenness, no matter the situation, *except for work.* I never drank while I was at work; but from 5 p.m. to 1 a.m., I was drinking. While at work, I would routinely go through the shakes due to alcohol withdrawal.

Helene, a co-worker, invited me to a party in her neighborhood. This was about a decade after I got my two DUIs. I stopped by my place first, knocked back a couple of shots of vodka, grabbed a fresh liter, and drove to her house. People were hanging out in the street when I got there and a guy offered us a hit of weed. Helene said, *No thanks, we have work tomorrow.* I said, *Sure, why not?* So now I was drunk *and* high.

Around ten o'clock, Helene said she was going to bed and offered me her couch. I was totally wasted at this point and said, *Okay, thanks.* When she stepped into the bathroom, I snuck out of the house. As I walked to my car, people were looking at me and calling out, "Where you going, man? This isn't a good idea, man," but I kept walking, got in my car, and drove off.

I could not function. At the first intersection, I went through a red light, missed a turn, and flew straight into a six-foot ditch. I passed out for a few seconds, and when I awoke, shifted furiously back and forth from drive to reverse, but the car wouldn't budge. I was banged up but not badly hurt. I managed to climb out of the car and up the embankment; then I walked to a church across the street, tossing my keys into the bushes on the way.

Under Florida law, the cops can't arrest someone without proof that they'd been driving; and they wouldn't have proof *if I didn't have the keys.* After a few minutes, I walked across the street to a gas station, where I sat down on the ground. Two squad cars pulled up to the ditch and the cops got out and inspected the wreck. They looked around, saw me sitting there, and walked over. All my stuff was in the car, including my ID, and they were holding that and the registration, which they'd pulled out of the glove box.

"Mr. Kruse?" they asked. "What happened?"

"It's miracle we weren't killed," I said. "My friend was driving and the next thing I knew, we were in the ditch, and by the time I got out, he'd run off with my keys." I truly was a high-functioning drunk. They were staring at me. One of them got in my face.

"Come on! Man up! There's no friend."

"There is, there is! He ran off! I'm totally wasted." That last part was true. Otherwise, it was pure lies, and they knew it. But without a witness to say I'd been driving, and without the keys, they could not arrest me. They ran my record, but because my DUIs were from another state, they didn't show up. The cops called a tow truck for the car, told me to call a friend to come get me, and they drove off.

I called in sick the next morning. The phone rang and it was Helene, asking if I was okay. One of her neighbors had gone out for more beer and seen my car in the ditch. I told her, *Yeah, I'm fine*, and I'd see her tomorrow.

I thought I'd gotten away with murder, but the truth was, I'd gotten away *without* murder. At the very least, I could have gotten a third DUI, gone to prison, and had my license suspended for life. It wasn't until two years later, when I went to rehab, that I realized what really happened that night. I could have killed or maimed myself or someone else, ruined my own life or someone else's, but God gave me a second chance. I believe most humans believe in something: the sun; the moon; Buddha; God. When I chose Recovery, I had to choose a higher power, and I chose God. I know now that it was by the grace of God, who let me live that night, that I was able to face reality and accept the truth of my life.

Rx

But right now, I was miserable. After a time, I couldn't function, so I quit my job in 2011 and moved back to Jacksonville. A few months later, I found out that my old boss, drunk at the time, had died in a motorcycle accident. Crazy.

I went to work at yet another insurance agency. I didn't know it at the time, but all of this running away and moving around is called a geographical fix. I was making my life so shitty at one place that I thought moving and starting someplace new would fix the problem; but it didn't. The last place I worked I hated my boss.

She was terrible, paid me the minimum amount, and worked me to the bone. I always had to be on the phone so I figured out a way to call a disconnected telephone number and turn the volume down on the phone. So as the message would say *this number is no longer in service* over and over and over in my ear, I would make up a fake conversation. I actually would do this repeatedly, so I wouldn't have to talk to a real human and try and sell them insurance. Also, it would sound like I was working really hard so my boss would get off my ass. It was crazy behavior, but it worked. With my ridiculous wages, I barely got by, so much so that my diet would consist of a pizza and a bottle of booze for breakfast, lunch, and dinner, day in and day out for months.

Rx

It was December that year when I hit rock bottom. The annual tradition with my brother and his family was Christmas Eve dinner at his house. We'd all open gifts Christmas morning.

I showed up to Blaine's house this particular Christmas Eve extremely drunk with a bottle of vodka in tow. I was a mess and pretty much blacked out at this time. I got in his car with his wife in the front seat, and me with my niece and nephew in the back. I was acting silly and then started to mouth off at Blaine's wife. By the time we got to his in-laws house, he let the kids and his wife out of the car but told me stay. He closed his door and said to me that he would not allow me into their house in my condition and drove me to my buddy Vince's house down the street. I was so angry with Blaine, I slammed his car door when he dropped me off. Vince was with his family at the time but gave me his garage door code, so I went in and started drinking his beer. He told me to call a cab and be gone in an hour. So I did and waited for the cab to pick me up.

I went home, furious at Blaine, and slammed a bottle of vodka down, passed out, and woke up Christmas Day. I was so hungover, but filled with so much shame about how I acted, that I just started drinking again. I puked but kept going and going. Drinking and drinking. I was close to killing myself at this point.

The next few weeks were the worst of my life. I had lost most of my family and the few friends I had left. I was alone and depressed. I didn't want to go on anymore.

22

> *I recover out loud*
> *when others can't.*

22

In January 2012, I was a razor's edge away from being homeless. I looked at myself in the mirror and said *I'm ready to die*. I was so sick, *and tired of being sick and tired*, I was at the end of my rope. I felt as if I were already dead in so many ways. I said aloud to my reflection, "Nate, you're going to die." It rushed at me like an oncoming train. The constant chase for my next bout of drunkenness, resenting every one, and disappointing the people I loved became overwhelming. That is when God intervened and gave me enough humility and strength to call the only person I knew would pick up.

Alcoholism is not contagious, but recovery is.

—Nan Robertson

Everything in life begins with one step. The biggest step for me was to feel safe enough to reach out to someone and admit I couldn't go on any more, admit I was out of control and didn't know what to do or where to go. I had to feel safe enough to tell someone I was fucked and needed help. When I felt I could do that, I called my mother, Caroline. I told her I needed help.

She is the one person who has always stood by me. There were times when she couldn't, because she couldn't stand up for herself. I get that. But when other people gave up on me or just plain didn't care, my mom was always there; which is pretty remarkable when you consider what I've put her through.

Mom said, "Give me a couple of hours and I'll call you back with options." She did. She consulted with Annie, the Marketing Manager at Pine Grove, and between them, they recommended a California rehab center near the beach or one in the mountains of Utah. I'd loved mountains ever since I was a little kid, so I chose Utah. Annie was instrumental in getting me into Cirque Lodge. It was located at the bottom of Provo Canyon in the serenity of the mountains with the Sundance Ski Resort nearby with a second facility; it was amazing. The whole place was designed to help people like me overcome addictions and co-occurring disorders. Their claim is they treat people with alcohol and drug addictions in an atmosphere of "kindness, dignity, and respect."

I quit my job the next day and notified the landlord I was breaking my lease. When I decided to check myself into rehab my Mom came all the way out from Mississippi to pick up Justappear and take him back to her farm.

Vince helped me pack my stuff into one of those storage containers, which was no fun because something was seriously wrong with my back (I'd already had two surgeries and would have two more before the problem was eventually solved). I didn't let it stop me, though; I'd turned a corner and there was no going back.

But it didn't stop me from drinking, either. My thinking was, I'm never going to drink again once I get to rehab, so let me drink as much as I can now. I was even drunk for my phone interview with Cirque's clinical director. I was at a neighbor's house, eight beers in, when my cell phone rang with an Orem area code, so I knew it was her. I grabbed two fresh cans, ran out to my Jeep, put her on speakerphone, and sat there with a beer in each hand telling her how committed I was to getting sober. At one point she asked, "Do you need to go into detox first?" I said No: detox would cost a lot more money.

"Okay," she said, "but, if you're currently drinking"—she didn't know how currently I was drinking—"I suggest you do a step-down and drink less and less over the next four days until you get here, or you'll have to go into detox." "No, no," I told her. "I'll do the step-down. That sounds good."

What sounded better was to keep on drinking, which was what I did over the next three days. I spent my last night in Florida at Vince's place. He was going to drive me to the airport in the morning after a ceremonial daybreak shot of vodka, but it turned out he had to work that day, so another friend swung by to give me a lift.

I thought, Okay, I'll have a drink on my layover in Atlanta. But my next flight was already boarding when I got there, so I couldn't stop at the bar. No problem, I told myself. I'll have a cocktail on the plane. When the drinks cart came by, I whipped out a twenty. "I'm sorry, sir," the flight attendant said, "it's credit card only." I had five cards, but they were mostly maxed out and the embarrassment of having them rejected was too much to contemplate, so I didn't drink on the plane, either. I thought, Man, I've got the worst luck ever.

At least when we touched down in Salt Lake City, I was able to walk off the plane. There had been a distant possibility of me needing a wheelchair . . ..

23

*The most powerful person
in the room
is the person
without anything
to hide.*

23

Addiction is an illness, a disease, an ailment . . . you'll find all kinds of definitions. But it's really an affliction. Something that causes actual pain and suffering of all sorts. And it's widespread. It can be nicotine, cocaine, overeating; for me it was alcohol. For Mom, it was Tom. He was her drug of choice, her addiction. And for Tom, it was sex, power, and money.

I was so emotionally and physically, dismantled, I had no idea what to do, where to turn, how to move forward.

If I could have gone back in time, my first inclination would have been to fix things, but there was nothing I could do. I remembered Mom sobbing. I couldn't stop Tom from being an asshole; I couldn't even talk to him because I remembered how he beat the crap out of me.

The one thing I could do was drink. I pickled myself in vodka from the time I was 17 until I was 34. Now it was time to change for good.

A lot of guys have their first drink as a kid, but unlike them, I didn't know when to stop. I didn't want to stop, mostly because being drunk made me forget about everything that was bothering me. Tom had little use for me other than as a target. Blaine was the good son, and I was "chubs," the dummy, the screwup. Tom did things that stayed with me forever. He liked telling me what a screw-up I was, and it didn't stop with words. He beat me with a belt and sometimes with a switch that I had to choose from a tree branch. He also had a wooden paddle he'd made and stained right in front of Blaine and me that he would hit us with. The man was sadistic in his discipline.

I discovered that a huge part of my Recovery was going to be about him and that shook me. The last thing I wanted was to even think about him.

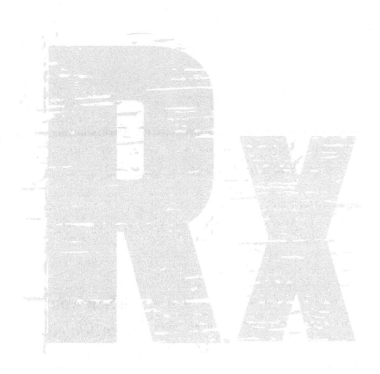

24

*Where your
attention goes,
your energy flows.*

24

February 27, 2012 is my official sobriety date. A sobriety date is commonly referred to as a birthday, and this was the day I was born into a wonderful thing called *Recovery*.

I walked off the plane in Salt Lake City about 10 p.m. and was descending the escalator to the baggage claim area. To my surprise, there was a man holding a sign with my name on it!

I remember I was chatting with a couple from the flight, and when they saw me walk up to him, they said "Wow! We didn't know you were such a big shot." I felt like a big shot because that had never happened to me before. His name was Kevin, and he was picking me up to drive me straight to Cirque. He was so nice; he told me everything would be alright. We retrieved my suitcase and headed to his car.

Salt Lake was experiencing what seemed, to me, like a super blizzard snowstorm, but was probably just normal for the locals. I felt like a little kid walking in the snow for the first time in a long time. We drove about an hour south to north Orem, just at the bottom of Provo Canyon where Cirque Lodge is located. We drove through the arched stone entrance. Kevin dropped me off at the front doors and asked me to wait there while he parked, and he would take me inside.

I lit up a smoke and looked around at the calm silent snowfall. I saw the outline of the massive Wasatch mountain range, Mt. Timpanogos, over 11,000, feet just to the north and Y Mountain to the south. Looking inside the doors, I saw a receptionist and a few people walking through. I quietly said to myself, "Nate, how the hell did you end up here?"

I felt fear, consternation, apprehension, but also excitement, as if I were on an adventure. I didn't have to go to work in the morning and do all the shit I hated doing. I was at this mysterious place where I had no expectations and no idea what was about to occur.

Kevin told me to follow him, and we went inside. Large, comfortable leather couches and chairs in Native American motifs, wooden tables, soft lighting, all reflecting an inviting warmth.

It was 11 p.m. and quiet inside. The receptionist was really sweet. She had me sign in, and then I was escorted to the second floor where I checked in. At this point, Kevin gave me a hug and wished me the best. The night manager, Amy, had me fill out some paperwork and told me to breathe in the breathalyzer. I was so glad I hadn't had a drink on the plane or in the bar at the airport. For some reason, God did not allow me to drink this day. I passed.

Amy gave me a cup and I followed a staff member into the bathroom to take the first of many urinalysis tests during my stay. Once again, I passed, and thus was officially admitted into the very place where I would learn the most inspiring, important, and profound information of my adult life.

I was taken to my room where there were four beds. One bed had a guy sleeping in it and the other three were empty. I chose the best one, closest to the door. Subconsciously I figured if I needed to leave, I wasn't far from the exit.

The staff went through my suitcase and bag looking for any alcohol or drugs. Then they said to get some rest as I would have a very busy day ahead of me to go through my paperwork and get processed. I went out back and smoked one more time. When I returned to the room and was alone (with the exception of my sleeping roommate), I just sat on the edge of my bed pondering what was in store for my future for the next two months. I laid down but it took me awhile before I could go to sleep.

The next morning, I got up at 6 a.m. and had the chance to meet my new roommate Brian. He had just been released from prison where he spent a few years due to heroin-related offenses. He seemed like a nice guy. It was his fourth rehab stint.

A staff member swung by our room and told us that breakfast was at 7 and we had an hour to eat. Brian and I went out back for a smoke and chatted a bit about ourselves. Then we went upstairs to the third floor to eat.

Cirque bought the quite famous, at least locally, Osmond Productions studio, an enormous facility where the Osmond family recorded their hit show from 1976 to 1979, *Donny & Marie*. They also had a very active commercial production department where many famous television commercials were recorded, including an entire series of *Wheaties* commercials with the "old" Bruce Jenner, none of which ever aired due to the cancellation of the Olympics for the US in 1980.

So this place, called the studio, was massive and could house fifty residents trying to get sober. Cirque also has another building further up the canyon near Robert Redford's *Sundance Ski Resort* that holds about ten residents and is more private.

We went to the third floor where I discovered a rather spectacular, huge dining room sporting floor to ceiling windows which revealed the amazing Mt. Timpanogos. The sun was literally bursting through them, breathtaking and so beautiful. It filled my heart with this magical feeling of safety and love.

About forty residents were in line sampling breakfast foods buffet-style—eggs, bacon, pancakes, fresh fruit, and pretty much any kind of breakfast food you could think of or hope for. The cooks were making special entrees on a massive cook top. I felt like I was at five-star hotel. Really.

Coffee was brewing and there were snack bars, cereals, and two huge refrigerators full of milks and cheeses. It was glorious. Most people kept to themselves or were sitting at tables with other residents. I met some people and enjoyed some light conversation. The men sat together and the women sat together—no co-mingling, it seemed. All fine by me.

I was just thinking to myself that less than five days ago I was on my last leg, about to give up on life, and now I was in this amazing setting eating the best food I had denied myself for so many years.

I finished and returned to the second floor where I met the man himself, the Director of Cirque. He knew my mom well from being in the recovery community. He came right up to me and introduced himself, giving me a big hug. It was like an acceptance kind of hug; like 'Nate, you are in the right place and are loved.' He was so positive, and the gratitude he was exuding was contagious. I've gotten to know him over the years, and he hasn't changed one bit. If I ever needed a role model in my life, this was the guy.

There was a large staff to handle all fifty residents. Things ran smoothly that first day and the process became clear. I needed to commit to them and do the work they gave me to understand this disease of alcoholism and addiction.

I, of course, didn't commit and pissed away the first few days I was there, but again, they accepted me and let me take my time.

I went through intake, which meant filling out a stack of forms, with ten other people. They gave each of us a copy of *The Big Book*, the bible of Alcoholics Anonymous (the Twelve Step program created by William Griffin Wilson and Robert Smith, MD, known in the recovery community as Bill W. and Dr. Bob). I tell people that I didn't even know how to spell AA when I arrived at Cirque. That was about to end. Our first homework assignment was to read 164 pages of *The Big Book*. It covered the first three steps. Then we had to fill out a series of worksheets that required an excessive amount of writing.

I opened the book and there were the steps, all twelve of them:

1. *We admitted we were powerless over alcohol—that our lives had become unmanageable.*

2. *Came to believe that a Power greater than ourselves could restore us to sanity.*

3. *Made a decision to turn our will and our lives over to the care of God as we understood Him.*

4. *Made a searching and fearless moral inventory of ourselves.*

5. *Admitted to God, to ourselves, and to another human being the exact nature of our wrongs.*

6. *Were entirely ready to have God remove all these defects of character.*

7. *Humbly asked Him to remove our shortcomings.*

8. *Made a list of all persons we had harmed, and became willing to make amends to them all.*

9. *Made direct amends to such people wherever possible, except when to do so would injure them or others.*

10. *Continued to take personal inventory and when we were wrong promptly admitted it.*

11. *Sought through prayer and meditation to improve our conscious contact with God as we understood Him, praying only for knowledge of His will for us and the power to carry that out.*

12. *Having had a spiritual awakening as the result of these steps, we tried to carry this message to alcoholics, and to practice these principles in all our affairs.*

Even the first three were more than I could deal with at that point. I thought, *I'm not good at this.* I was in a haze; my body was withdrawing from all the alcohol. It took me at least a month to dry out.

I set aside *The Big Book* and picked up the one Vince gave me as I was leaving. It was a memoir by Duff McKagan, the bass player from Guns N' Roses. It was about the ugly side of the band, about his abuse of vodka and cocaine and then getting sober and how he did it. I read it every night before I went to sleep. There was one scene I will never, ever forget, about when he'd drunk so much, he vomited all over the floor, and, desperate to maintain his high, tried to suck the vomit out of the carpet. The image was so repulsive, it made me shudder. At the same time, I understood why he did it. I thought of the time Vince and I had gone to an all-you-can-eat sushi place, and I shoved so much sushi down my throat (and vodka, of course), that I threw all of it up when I got home and sat staring at the mess, thinking, Dammit, Nate, you just wasted fifty bucks. That got to me, that I could actually get why someone would try to eat his own puke. I didn't have to actually do it; understanding it was enough.

That did it. I was all in. My mindset was, *I'm here, I'm doing this, I'm committed.* I have never looked back.

The fifth day I was in treatment, *the light turned on.* Things started clicking for me, and I just made the decision to dedicate all of my time and energy in this once-in-a-lifetime opportunity. It was as if I needed a few days for my body to get rid of the booze and the cloud to leave my head. I needed sleep and healthy food. Once I received those things, I was ready to rock 'n roll.

Cirque would schedule daily experiential hikes and walks in the mountains. This was where I learned how detrimental my smoking had become. I was hiking up those mountains and the crisp air cut my lungs; it was a pain like no other. The hike coordinator, Carey, was a mountain man and an amazing hiker. He tailed me and encouraged me to keep going no matter how long it took. He helped me so much.

That was the attitude of everyone at Cirque—love, encouragement, and lots of support. I dove into *The Big Book* of AA and learned all about the Twelve Steps and even had a sponsor to help me with the first three steps while I was there.

He was a nice fellow and took sobriety very seriously. I
followed his advice. I could see a positive change in me physically and mentally, but the spiritual part was what I really
needed to address.

Rx

About a month into my stay my therapist Bob and I went
on a walk-and-talk. Bob was a very calm and collected man
who really connected with me. He took me to the Provo River
and told me that since I had finished steps 1 and 2, now was
the time for step 3—turn my life and will over to the care of
my Higher Power.

I hadn't chosen a Higher Power yet; I could not acknowledge
there was something greater than me. But when we arrived at
this pristine river, rushing from all of the spring melt (it was
April), he told me to go sit by the river and think about my
choice; if nothing happened, then it was all good, but if I felt
something, then explore it.

Beside that rushing water, seeing the power of it drag-
ging limbs and rocks on its journey, the sound that drowned
out everything but my thoughts, I just closed my eyes. What
happened next was a spiritual awakening for me. I had cast
God out of my life years ago thinking He had cursed me
with all the negative shit that happened. But when I closed
my eyes, there was God waiting for me. It wasn't like a clear
image of Him, but a feeling that came over me. I could really hear the river rushing now and feel the wind blowing
through my hair. These physical feelings touched me in
such a way that *my mind and my heart were affected.* They were
opened in a way I had never felt before, and I knew He loved
me and would forgive me *always*, as long as I allow Him to.

This was a miraculous and pivotal moment in my life. It was like having an old friend you pissed off for so many years just love you unconditionally and hug you right when you needed it. That is how I felt about God. At that very second I prayed to the Lord asking Him for forgiveness of my ways and pleading with him to come back into my heart as my heavenly Father.

When I opened up my eyes, the sun was warm on my face, my therapist was about a hundred yards away sitting on a bench, and everything just seemed right with me. Suddenly I had a purpose again. It was as if I just made good with the most important person I could ever have in my life and He accepted me with open arms.

I can now, finally, turn things over to the care of God when my life gets sideways and know He has a plan for me and *it is not calamity*. I was truly born again, saved again, and ready to take my Recovery to a new level. I walked back up to Bob, and we looked at each other and smiled. We didn't have to say anything; we just hugged and celebrated the most profound experience of my life with love and a laugh.

25

*If it fits,
make it stick.
If it doesn't apply,
let it fly.*

25

was about four weeks into my two-month stay when I had a physician assistant, Nate, confront me about my smoking habit. As a resident, I was able to check in with a doctor once a week. Steve would take notes and help Dr. Mack out. He told me one time that I was there getting sober from booze, but I was still killing myself by smoking. I was very stubborn at first and said, "No way are you taking my cigarettes away from me." But another week went by, and Steve asked again why I was still smoking.

He noticed how much I had changed so far in my sobriety and said I should reconsider quitting smoking. I'd quit once before when I was thirty but that lasted about two months. This time, however, he said there was a stopping aid called Chantex. Other residents had some success with it, and Dr. Mack could prescribe it for me.

I thought about it later that night and said, *Fuck it, Nate. Just try to quit. This is your time!* So I went on Chantex for about a week. I was shocked that I was able to give my last pack of smokes away. But I was able to do it!

After two days, cigarettes began to taste different. Within a week, they tasted like chalk; in ten days, I gave my unopened packs away. I was dumbfounded: smoking tasted so nasty now, I didn't even want to light up. I haven't smoked since, which is not to say I don't remember how much I enjoyed it. I'm like a bloodhound: I can smell a cigarette downwind a mile away.

Sometimes it smells really good. Other times, I'll be shopping and walk by someone who must be living in a smoke-filled ten-by-ten box, and I'll almost gag and think, *Oh, that's so nasty—thank God I don't smoke anymore.*

I couldn't believe the gift Steve gave me by not giving up on me. I have been smoke-free since March of 2012, and I didn't think I would ever be able to quit that horrible habit. I am so grateful to Steve and Dr. Mack for saving my lungs and prolonging my life.

RX

I was in rehab one day, talking about the fight with Tom when I was 17.

"Listen, man," my therapist said, "you grew physically after that, and you grew mentally, but you did not grow *emotionally.*" I was taken aback when he said that; but it was true.

And here's something interesting. I was talking to Mom recently about that fight and *she didn't even remember it.* She didn't recall coming outside with the phone. She remembered telling me about Tom's cheating, and she remembered me storming out of the kitchen. But she said she thought we'd had the fight at his office and that it had ended there. She was actually *surprised* when I told her that we had been fighting viciously on the deck before she came out of the house. *She had to have heard us and seen it,* or why would she have gotten the phone and threatened to call the cops? Still, she had to be reminded that it had even happened.

Mom felt she may have repressed the memory because it was so terrible; the two people she loved most in the world seemingly trying to annihilate each other. I understand why she'd want to forget. I wanted to forget it, too, but I couldn't.

That fight on the deck was overwhelming. I don't think I've ever been so furious, so out of control. It was like my head exploded. Emotionally, I just shut down and stayed that way for seventeen years until I began my Recovery. Today, I *feel* my emotions, good and bad. They're mostly good, especially when I hold my daughter; I feel a love I didn't know was possible. There are times I feel anger, but I work on it, every day.

RX

I never knew what I'd put Mom through until I became sober. One day my therapist, said, "Let's talk about that failed intervention."

I said, "What? No, you must be mixing me up with someone else."

"Oh, no. Your mother told me about it. She was really worried about you." He went on to say that around six months before . . ..

> My mom had called Tom and my brother. That was when the three of us were living in Jacksonville and she had come for a visit. I was drinking and smoking a lot at that point. I never hid anything; I didn't think I had a problem, so why should I hide?
>
> Well, she took one look at me and could see how bad off I was. She called Blaine and Tom and told them that she believed I was an alcoholic, and that they should stage an intervention and get me some help. Tom said, "Nah, there's nothing wrong with Nate; he's fine; he can handle it." And he refused to help. So she went back to home and continued to pray.
>
> Later I was hanging out with Blaine, and I was really drunk, when he told me, "Oh, yeah, Mom called me. She thinks you're an alcoholic and tried to get me and Tom to do an intervention with you."

I couldn't believe it! Blaine said, "Yeah, she sure did."
"Bullshit! I'm calling her right now!" And I called her.

When this attempted interaction did not materialize, I did not drink to be social. I did not drink to get woozy, or even to get drunk. I drank to get fucked up, period. I drank to the point I couldn't even walk. When I couldn't walk anymore, that's how I knew I was drunk. Then I drank until I blacked out. That's how I was when Blaine told me this—in a blackout state. Only I wasn't asleep. I was awake; awake and saying and doing shit. Even as I tell this story, I have no cognizant memory of it. None. It's like it never happened. And here's my therapist, who I trust, telling me, "Yeah, it happened."

It must have been really late when Blaine originally told me this, well past midnight, but at the time, I called Mom anyway and she picked up the phone because she always takes my calls. She said, "Hello, Nate, are you okay?" And I laid into her. I mean, I cussed her out—my own mother. I had never, ever spoken to her this way, but I did then. I don't know what I said because I don't remember any of it.

Now I was at Cirque, newly sober, and my therapist was telling me I had treated my mother this badly over the phone. I said, "That's bullshit! You're lying to me! If I'd done that, I would know." And he said, "Call her now. Ask her yourself." When he said that, I knew it was true.

The truth matters. And the truth was, my mother was right. I had been just barely hanging on, making really bad decisions; driving drunk; doing coke just to stay awake enough to drink more vodka all weekend long, week after week. That was my life.

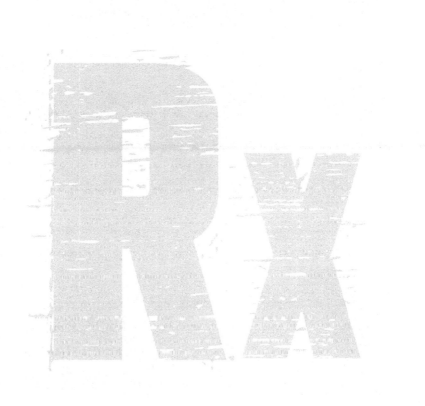

26

*Don't forget
why you started.*

26

D r. Bob, one of the co-founders of Alcoholics Anonymous, was a physician in Akron, Ohio, who became sober on June 10, 1935 and remained sober until his death from colon cancer in 1950. In his book, *The Big Book*, he wrote a prescription for alcoholics and it included these three things:

R. H. SMITH, M. D.
2ND NATIONAL BLDG.   AKRON, OHIO
TELEPHONE: HE 8588   REG. NO.

℞   FOR_____ alcoholics
     ADDRESS_____DATE____ Feb 1937

Always remember it
     1. Trust God
     2. Clean house
     3. Help others

NR | 1 | 2 | 3 | INF.   M. D.

In his lifetime, he helped over 5,000 people become sober. His prescription for sobriety was simple. Only it's not simple *unless you follow it every day*. If you don't, it will seem impossible to catch up.

What works for me is to trust the process for the moment. For today only. I can't promise that I'll never drink again, but I can promise I won't drink today: that, I can swear to. I can handle the next 24 hours. If I'm not able to do that, I focus on one thing at a time. When it's time to meditate, I put my phone in silent mode. When I do that, my meditation is better, my work is better, and I can go throughout my day.

This is how I keep sober, how I maintain my sanity. It takes maintenance, persistence, and practice.

The days at Cirque were repetitive but new at the same time. We woke up and ate at the same time, did our hikes or equine therapy at the same time, and had our process groups at the same time. They kept asking us to do more and more difficult exercises and really stick our necks out to reach those hard feelings and eradicate them once and for all. What I remember most is how uncomfortable I felt, finally reaching the source of my disease of addiction and alcoholism. They gave me a safe place to face it and move forward without it.

Rx

Part of the program at Cirque was giving back to the community, and the second week I was there, I spent a day at a local thrift store cleaning up donated appliances so they could be put on sale. We were allowed to look around afterward, and I bought myself a hard-sided Samsonite briefcase, the kind with metal flip-up locks on top and compartments inside. It was old and stained and perfect. It supported my going-to-work mentality: I filled it with *The Big Book*, a printout of the Twelve Steps, pens and papers, and everything else I needed to do the work of Recovery. Some residents thought it was goofy and told me so, but I didn't care. My only job now was getting sober, and my briefcase was a symbol of that.

After a week or so, a resident suggested I stop shaving and grow a sobriety beard. I liked the idea. As my beard came in and got longer, so did the length of my sobriety.

Those first weeks were an education. I met a woman, another resident, and felt a spark. She had a history of drug use and prostitution and had attempted suicide more than once. I felt sorry for her and wanted to help. Cirque was careful about keeping women and men apart most of the time, but we chatted when we could and passed notes to each other about what music and movies we liked.

The next day my counselor said he wanted to talk to me. He sat me down in his office with three other counselors and they told me to cool it with this woman. My walls went up. I told them they had it all wrong. I wasn't remotely interested in having sex with her, I knew she was having a hard time, and I just wanted to be a friend.

"Just listen for a minute," they said. They explained that each patient was there for a reason, and I couldn't know how my words were affecting her process, her ability to heal. "She may want more than words from you," one of them said. "She may want to use you as a distraction from the work she has to do on herself." They told me to stop focusing on her so both she and I could focus on ourselves and the reasons we were there. It was hard for me to hear and accept, but once I did, it made sense. I kept my distance after that.

The Twelve Steps took a while to make sense to me, but I finally got the hang of them in my second week. The first thing I noticed was that the Steps are written as "we," not "I," the idea being that it's a fellowship, you're not alone, we're all in this together. There's strength in knowing there are others who are fighting the same demons you are, and who are committed to help you fight your demons just as you're committed to helping them fight theirs.

The next thing I noticed was that the heart of the Steps is about taking responsibility for your life and not blaming

anyone else for the hole you had dug for yourself. The reason
I was at Cirque to begin with was that I was full of excuses: I had bad luck, everyone was against me, my father was a
creep. Even after I got to rehab, I was still making excuses,
like refusing to start reading *The Big Book* until I'd finished
the McKagan one.

At Cirque, when we were finished with an AA or cocaine
anonymous meeting, we would stand in a circle, put our right
foot inside, and say the serenity prayer.

> *God, grant me the serenity*
>
> *To accept the things I cannot change;*
>
> *Courage to change the things I can;*
>
> *And wisdom to know the difference.*

Putting one foot in was to symbolize a foundation for
our healing and the maintenance program for when we left
Cirque and were on our own. It makes sense. I still do it now
when I go to other meetings. I want to go through the entire
process to make it happen for myself in my everyday life. It
might look strange to other people, but it makes sense to me,
and so I do it.

RX

There are a few events at Cirque where residents may in-
vite their families to come for a visit and participate in ther-
apeutic sessions with them. The big deal event was called
The Ring of Fire. Mom came to work with me. Tom was now
in jail; and Blaine was doing his best to provide for and raise
his family; and it was time for *my* Ring of Fire.

I'd been an observer at many of these and never once did
I see a family member say they were sorry for something. It
was always the other way around.

The Ring of Fire is an exercise where a number of families sit in a circle, while one family sits in the middle to do major therapy work for everyone to observe. Talk about hard and embarrassing! But my therapist and another therapist were inside the ring with my mom and me. They assured us that this was the time to exorcise the demons. I knew it was coming as I had seen other residents go through it; but it was way different now, *being inside the Ring.*

Around 20 residents and their families sat in a circle with my mom and me in the center, sitting and facing each other. With us were two therapists leading the exercise. One of them started by saying, "Nate, I want you to ask your mother, 'Mom, how did my addiction affect you?'"

Whatever my mom said, I'd repeat back to her. The point of the Ring of Fire was to provide a safe space for addicts and their loved ones to talk to one another. Making me repeat my mom's words was a way to ensure that what I heard was what she said, and for her to know that she was being heard. So I asked my mom how my addiction affected her, and she said she lived in constant fear that I was going to die. I repeated that back to her exactly, and she said, "Yes, that's what I said."

But then she went off script and started telling me how she felt she'd wronged *me.*

"Nate, I want you to know that I've been a terrible mother to you."

"Mom, you're not supposed to say that!"

But she felt so much guilt, and the therapist saw what was going on, so he allowed it to continue. She cried and told me how sorry she was for all the things she did wrong, and then I looked into her eyes and told her I forgave her. That made her cry more, but in a good way. And then she forgave me for everything I had put her through.

My therapist put a garbage can next to my mom and I told her that was called the Shilt Bucket where you throw away all of the tissues we were going to use. Shilt stood for Shame and Guilt and Bob said that we would go through a lot of it.

It was excruciating for both of us, but we were committed to doing the hard work. Then came time to face the biggest issue and that was Tom. Bob placed us side by side in chairs, then placed an empty chair in front of us. That is where Tom would have been seated, had he been there. This was a defining moment for both of us as this was our chance to tell Tom all the shit he had done to hurt us. And we let him have it! We didn't hold anything back because we knew this was the time to speak about the hurt he dished out to us over all the years, but also the time to take our power back! We went wild. I was shouting, "How dare you do this to me? How dare you cheat on my mother? How dare you *steal* my money?" Mom was screaming too. It was something to behold.

After doing this, all of the people around the circle were crying with us. It was cathartic and real and brutal but it felt amazing. At the end, Bob had my mom and me forgive Tom, not for him, but for us to move forward without the anger and resentment. This was such a powerful step in my Recovery evolution. We each forgave Tom; then Bob told us to go take a break as we were officially done with the Ring of Fire exercise.

Leave it to my mom, though, as she asked in front of everyone if we could move Tom's chair outside. Bob said sure with a smile. Mom and I took the chair that represented Tom (it was one of those plastic ones) outside, and then we both looked at each other and proceeded to kick the living shit out of it!

We stomped and crushed that chair to nothing and said aloud that Tom had no more power over us, and he would never hurt us again. That was it! That was the final time I ever felt that he could hurt me. No more. I was now fully responsible for my actions moving forward. It was awesome and to do it with Mom, who had been hurt so much by Tom, was a blessing. Thank you, Cirque for allowing my mother and me to live life without that tyrant any longer!

We kicked it, trampled it, mutilated it, stomped on it. We destroyed that chair. It lay on the ground in pieces, and we were standing there, staring at it, panting from the exertion. After this fairly violent experience, suddenly here came the marketing director with a prospective family, giving them a tour of the grounds. "Oh," she said with a bright smile, "I guess we've had some furniture damage." She saw a busted chair, but we saw victory. We faced the demon, we faced the fear, we faced it all. And we came through.

RX

There was a room where we'd meet for group therapy sessions and on the wall were a couple of posters, one with The Twelve Steps and another with The Twelve Traditions, which are ways of reading into and beyond the Steps. Here are the Traditions:

1 *Our common welfare should come first; personal recovery depends upon AA unity.*

2. *For our group purpose there is but one ultimate authority—a loving God as He may express Himself in our group conscience. Our leaders are but trusted servants; they do not govern.*

3. *The only requirement for AA membership is a desire to stop drinking.*

4. *Each group should be autonomous except in matters affecting other groups or AA as a whole.*

5. *Each group has but one primary purpose—to carry its message to the alcoholic who still suffers.*

6. *An AA group ought never endorse, finance, or lend the AA name to any related facility or outside enterprise, lest problems of money, property, and prestige divert us from our primary purpose.*

7. *Every AA group ought to be fully self-supporting, declining outside contributions.*

8. *Alcoholics Anonymous should remain forever nonprofessional, but our service centers may employ special workers.*

9. *AA, as such, ought never be organized; but we may create service boards or committees directly responsible to those they serve.*

10. *Alcoholics Anonymous has no opinion on outside issues; hence the AA name ought never be drawn into public controversy.*

11. *Our public relations policy is based on attraction rather than promotion; we need always maintain personal anonymity at the level of press, radio, and films.*

12. *Anonymity is the spiritual foundation of all our traditions, ever reminding us to place principles before personalities.*

The Twelve Traditions of Alcoholics Anonymous at
https://www.aa.org/assets/en_US/smf-122_en.pdf, accessed July 23, 2019

I studied the posters to figure out what they meant and how they spoke to me; and what leapt out was the idea of at-

traction rather than promotion. It comes from the very be-
ginnings of AA when Bill W. would gather drunks off the
street, drag them to his house, and, with the help of his wife
Lois, sober them up with endless pots of black coffee and
preach the gospel of how he became sober in the hope of inspiring them to become sober too. They'd spend the night at
the house, awake sober the next morning, and then go back
out and get drunk all over again. Bill W. had to learn, just as
I did, that we're not here to save anyone. We're not here to
talk anyone into sobriety. We're not here to say, "You've got
to do this because it's noon, and you're lying there wasted on
a park bench." What we're here to do is attract others by our
own behaviors, actions, and choices, by setting an example
of what sobriety looks like and sounds like, and not by trying
to sell it with promises of how great it will be.

It is great, but you can only get there if you take responsibility for your life and decide that you want to get better.
My mom tells a story of a couple who had been at each other's
throats for years. They had a bunch of kids, and now the wife
was dying of cancer. The husband called my mom, weeping,
and asked her to come and help them make peace with each
other while there was still time. So she went to their house
and the wife was propped up on a sofa, and everything my
mom tried to do to bring them together, the wife rejected. She could barely sit up, and what little energy she had,
she used for rage. She did not want things to get better; she
wanted everyone to know how angry she was. She died without ever making peace with her husband.

You're wasting your time if someone doesn't want to change,
even if that someone is you. But once you make that decision

and commit to change, there is nothing and no one who can stop you.

My journey to sobriety started with alcohol as my god. They call it spirits for a reason, and I was worshiping the spirit of vodka. The journey continued as I learned that sobriety is just the beginning. The hard work comes next. It's called Recovery. The therapy started. The anxiety started. The depression started. All the crap I'd been pushing down inside me started to surface, and it hurt. Inside I was shouting, *Wait a second! I got sober for this?* But by discovering who I was, honoring the self I found, and learning to put my own well-being first, I was living the dream.

People would say to me, "Nate, I can't believe you're never going to drink again." And I tell them, "Whoa! I never said that." It's not like I went into rehab and signed a lifetime agreement saying, "I will never smoke another cigarette or another joint, or snort another line, or have another drink." I would never make a promise like that; even the thought of it makes me anxious. What I tell people is, "I'm doing this for *today only.* I will not drink alcohol *today.* I will not smoke a cigarette *today.* I will not smoke a joint or snort cocaine *today.* For all I know, I'll have a drink next year, next month, next week. I can't predict how well I'll be able to manage myself in the future. But I can promise to control myself now, in the moment, *today.*"

It's not that I don't want to drink; I wish I could. But, as I have said for years, drinking makes me break out into handcuffs, and I begin making extremely bad decisions. I will repeat: I am an alcoholic; that is a fact. It is also a fact that I cannot drink like normal human beings, because once I start, I cannot stop. This is what I know. This is black and white for me. There is no in-between, no gray area. If I take one sip of vodka, I'll move on to a double, and then five more doubles; then I'll finish the bottle, and make my way to a liquor store for another. There's no end to my drinking. I cannot stop.

That's why I see things in terms of black and white. There's a right way and a wrong way in my world. There are no more gray areas for me, no more pushing the limits until they break. I do what I need to do and stay in my lane. That's my Recovery program. There's no going to a bar for me because a bar is a gray area. I know I won't be forced to drink there, but if I'm in a place where alcohol is the main thing they serve, the potential is high that I'll have a drink. If I don't go there, the potential is zero. That's black and white.

It's the same with cigarettes; there's no middle ground. I used to smoke all the time; I couldn't imagine drinking without a cigarette in my hand, so I kept packs and lighters all over the place—in my pockets, my jacket, my car. I arrived at Cirque with four cartons. They let you smoke there; there's just so much they can ask you to give up at once. But they helped me eliminate that addiction from my life too.

RX

When I was settled in at Cirque and really kicking ass with the treatment, I was getting excited to know some of my fellow residents. I still have a strong relationship with some of these wonderful people, and I am grateful to God that they are on the journey with me.

One special man was John, and he was in my process group. He and I shared the love of getting dirty and doing our work that was needed to succeed in Recovery. He spoke his truth and didn't hold back, which I admired. He and I also shared our DOC (drug of choice) which was alcohol, so we clicked and supported each other from the jump.

What was great about John was that he also loved to laugh and have fun, something I thought we didn't get to do in rehab, *but shit, he had a knack to make you laugh!* We supported one another during these hard times by accepting our faults but also trusting the journey and knowing we were there in rehab for a reason, and that was *to get better.*

Another wonderful person I got to know and admired greatly was JoAnn. She was a sweet soul and like all of us came to Cirque broken. But I had the pleasure of watching her regain her strength and perspective on life. I fellowshipped with her at meetings and again, the love and support we shared was amazing. I am so proud of her and John and what they have accomplished and how amazing their lives are now by staying sober. It was bittersweet saying goodbye to all of these good people who made such a difference in my life.

Rx

When I left Cirque and moved in with my mom in May 2012, I was reunited with Justappear, and it was so great to squeeze that little boy again. I was able to be his Dad, sober now, and it was so much fun spending time with him. Unfortunately, God called Justappear up to heaven only a few months later. I was so sad and felt I lost a best friend, but my Recovery was teaching me that everything has a purpose and I should grieve his loss, but also honor him for helping to save me. I later named my *Ebay* store *JustAppear Retro* after him so that way he will always be a part of my life.

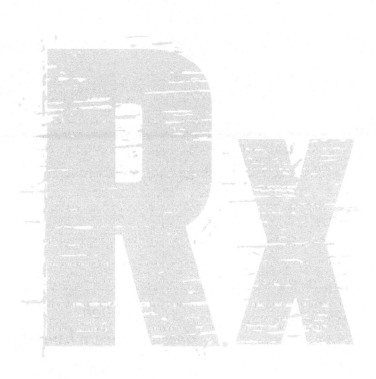

21

"A lion
doesn't concern himself
with the
opinions of sheep.

27

When I decided to move to Utah full time in September 2012, I was seven months sober and wanted to be closest to Cirque and the people with whom I became sober. I didn't have a job at the time and was just trying to stay away from bars and places that might mess with my new lifestyle. One of my good friends, Rick, and I were hanging out at Starbucks, and since we didn't have a lot of money, we decided to check out a thrift store nearby. I remembered the good experiences I had when we were doing our "giving back" activities and had the chance to venture into one of these establishments.

Rick took me to one called *Deseret Industries* in Provo. Boy, was I in for a surprise! I only knew of tiny little thrifts in Florida that smelled like a dingy old closet, but this place was the size of a *Walmart* and full of everything you could imagine! We were in the men's department and picked up this old baby blue Lacoste cardigan from the 1970s. It was in great shape and I said to Rick, "Don't you think someone would want this for more than the $3 I can buy it for?"

That is the exact time when God hit me over the head, and I woke up and said to myself, *Look around you, Nate. Look at all of this inventory; you can buy and sell these clothes and make a living at it.* I knew of *EBay* but had never used it. I didn't even know *PayPal* existed, let alone how to combine the two platforms to create the foundation of a business.

But in November 2012, I began the journey of becoming an *EBay* seller and opened *Justappear Retro* for business. I had never owned my own business, but I knew I could make other people rich, so why not me? I had a lot of motivation and time on my hands and gave this business all my attention and energy. I loved doing the research of what sold and what didn't and just made lists of brand names to hunt for. I made a lot of mistakes, but I allowed myself to do it and knew I would eventually find success.

When I began learning at Cirque about giving back and helping others, the thrift store work really made an impression on me; in fact, I thank God for thrift stores. I run an Internet retail business where I sell vintage clothes, boots, and accessories, mostly for men. And I love it, absolutely love it. It's the *finder* in me, the little kid who found my mom's diamond bracelet. I found him again when I went into Recovery. As the alcohol drained out of my body and my emotions resurfaced, I discovered my inner child and luckily, he still had a heartbeat. And it speeds up whenever I spot something that I know is quality goods and that I'll be able to sell to someone who would be thrilled to have it. It's the event of discovery that sparks my passion, like combing the beach with a metal detector. *How fun is that?* It's become a kind of addiction, but a good one. It supports me and my family and also my spirit, sometimes in ways I wouldn't expect.

I used to run into this woman at one of my regular stops. She was hard-nosed, aggressive, and rather rude. I'd be looking through a cart of new inventory, and she'd push me out of the way to get in there. I found it so annoying, I was about to tell her off one time, but something stopped me. I thought, Hold on; you don't know what she's going through. Why don't you just turn around and say good morning? I don't know where it came from, but I believe it was God. So I said, "Hey there, I'm Nathan. I've been seeing you around for years; I just wanted to introduce myself. I hope you're having a good morning."

She said, "I'm Aggie, and you know what? I'm not having a good morning. But it is what it is."

I said, "Well, if I can find a little bit of *gratitude* in something, that changes my morning."

"Oh, yeah, gratitude," she said, "that's what I'm working on now."

"Really? Why?"

"I don't know if I should say anything because people spread rumors. But, I just got sober two months ago."

"You're sober two months now? That's amazing! I'm four years sober."

"Wow! Really? That's great."

I told her about my business and how much I love treasure-hunting in thrift stores.

"Gee," she said, "I never looked at it that way. I just looked at it as a job. I'm so jaded; I hate everyone in here, and I hate doing this. I hate looking for stuff, and I hate reselling it. But I don't want to work for seven bucks an hour at a fast food place when I can make twenty bucks selling something."

I told her I'd sold insurance for a lot more than that, and it almost put me in the ground; and how grateful I was to be doing this. "Look at us," I said. "It's eleven-thirty in the morning on a Wednesday, and we're having a conversation. We don't have a time clock to punch; no one's looking over our shoulder and telling us to get back to work."

And she said, "You know, you're right."

We became friendly. Aggie is a few years sober now and we support each other. The best part for me is that she says our conversation changed her attitude. She smiles now, and I've even seen her talking to people. It's an awesome thing.

Truth to me is an action word. That's why I took a chance and started talking to Aggie. It's not enough to merely speak truth; I have to act truth. I felt God was telling me to reach out to this person. And it all came about in a thrift store, where unwanted things go for a second chance. Through my business, I get to give new life to things that people have discarded. And they're not always old. I find expensive, brand new things with the tags still on them, beautiful things. It's like a metaphor for my own life, which I came so close to discarding. I am resurrecting objects and giving them new meaning, much as Recovery resurrected me.

RX

It wasn't until about a year later when my mom suggested I hire someone to help get my inventory up for sale. Once I did that in January 2014, my business tripled in production, and I was on my way to financial freedom doing what I love which is thrifting and making my own money. God is amazing, and I am so grateful he inspired me to do this. I said it before, I am a finder at heart, and I get to fill my inner child's soul with what it loves the most—treasure hunting. I'm proud to say that my *EBay* thrifting business is still going strong after 7 years, and it's brought more blessings to my life than I could have ever have dreamed of.

RX

When it became time to leave Cirque, we were encouraged to stay away from things that may lead to a potential relapse. One of the things was to try and avoid getting into relationships for a year. I thought, man, that is rough but I took that advice to heart. It was hard and I was tested at first because Lizzy had called me when I was in Mississippi right after I moved there from Cirque and being freshly sober, she wanted to give our relationship another try, but I said no and rejected the idea since I felt I needed to learn how to stay sober and not complicate things with a relationship at this time.

She was very sad and confused but accepted my answer. She moved on and so did I. It wasn't until December of 2012 and I was ten months sober that God stepped in. I kept thinking about Lizzy and now that I had remained sober for almost a year, I felt it was the right time to call her. I texted her one fateful Sunday, and she wrote back saying that she couldn't talk then but would like chat later in the week.

I didn't want to take no for an answer so I asked again if she would talk now. She said yes but only if I didn't waste her time; still the same feisty Lizzy that I remembered from the Jacksonville days.

We spoke and caught up on what had been happening in our lives and what we wanted to do. After a few weeks of chatting, I offered her an opportunity to fly to Salt Lake City and go to a family week at Cirque to process our past and talk about the negative feelings, hoping for a brighter future. She took me up on that, and it was a very powerful week at Cirque working with my counselor and righting the wrongs. Another six months went by, but in June 2013, Lizzy made the decision to move to Utah permanently, and we started a new relationship with forgiveness and healing of the past and love filling the present moment.

RX

I was working my *EBay* business in Salt Lake, and everything seemed to be falling into place. Lizzy was back from Brooklyn, and we were on solid ground. But in 2014, I started experiencing some anxiety driving on the highway. I would get nervous going 70 mph and be thinking I may pass out from nerves and crash and kill myself. This was the same way I felt in Jacksonville. There it was—my anxiety was back haunting me. It became so bad over the next year that I just stopped driving the highways and took side streets everywhere, no matter how long it took me.

I was sober for two years, but the anxiety was holding me back again. I had to do something about it, and as my Recovery program would say, I needed to stop running from the hard things and face them.

I went to my therapist, and he knew what was happening. He told me that the anxiety was still plaguing me because I wasn't drinking anymore, so it kept raising its ugly head. He and I did a lot of work over the next few months retraining my brain to think differently, and with the aid of a non-narcotic SSRI medication called Paxil, I was able to overcome the anxiety. I still need to do daily and weekly maintenance but now have the tools to handle any flare-ups. This was a huge victory for me as it taught me that if there is anything in my life that holds me back, I can face it now and overcome it. *God is great.*

One morning in 2016, I received a call from a relative They started the conversation by telling me how sorry they were. I asked them, "Why are you sorry?"

They told me they just watched an episode of *American*

Greed on a major TV network and it was about Tom. I had no idea anyone would do an expose' on him of all people. There was a family photo of all of us, but *our* faces were blurred—not Tom's.

They went in detail about all the crazy shit Tom did; how he stole a bunch of money from unsuspecting people; how he tried hiring a hit-man to murder a key witness in his trial.

The past came crashing back; my body was flooded with negativity. I swore in that moment I would never watch that episode as it would only bring me anger and sadness. It was surely a trigger to drink as well. Here I am trying my best to build a life in Recovery, doing the next *right* thing, and *boom!* I get hit with this news. If I hadn't had a strong Recovery program, people whom I trust and rely on, and, of course, my Higher Power, I'm not sure I would have processed it in the right way. It was so key for me to know that none of the shit he did had anything to do with me.

28

*God has a plan.
Trust it,
live it,
enjoy it.*

28

There's a saying, "My politics are freedom, and my religion is love," which pretty much describes the values that govern my life now. The themes of freedom, love, and responsibility permeate The Twelve Steps and the Twelve Traditions, the foundation of my Recovery program, which evolved as my sobriety did. I honor the Twelve Traditions, but my allegiance is to my own program, which I think of as *The Roots of My Recovery* because they keep me stable and grounded. My Recovery is an ongoing journey and my program is too. As I learn new things about myself, I create new ways to grow my sobriety and sprout new roots to keep me planted in healthy soil. When I'm under stress or dealing with a thorny problem, I'm might feel tugged at and less grounded, but my roots hold me in place.

My Days of the Week:

Mindfulness Monday
Grati-Tuesday
Wellness Wednesday
Thoughtful Thursday
Freedom Friday
Social Saturday
Spiritual Sunday

MY RECOVERY ROOTS

1 Mindfulness

Mindfulness is simple: focus on now, right now, this very moment. Focus on where you are and what you are doing, not on what you did, or have to do, or are afraid you'll never do, or are afraid you *will do*. I don't like the term *meditate* because it implies action, whereas *mindfulness* is a way of *being*, a quieting of the mind so it can dwell in the present moment with you, wherever you are.

It enhances my sobriety by helping me disengage from anxiety-provoking thoughts, the very ones that used to drive me to drink. I used to obsess about my past, all the ways people had hurt me or I had hurt them, or all the things I'd done to sabotage my own well-being. When such thoughts come to me now, I think, *My past is my past; even yesterday is the past. It's there; I'll deal with it eventually. But now my focus is on feeding my daughter; or the cat; or preparing shipments; or cleaning the stove; or any of the everyday tasks that make up a life.*

Mindfulness helps my business by enabling me to function efficiently even when I'm under stress. I once got a nasty email from a customer demanding a refund because the shirt he bought was too small. That really got me going because I provide four measurements of every shirt I sell: chest, sleeve-length, shoulder to shoulder across the back, and length from collar to hem. I also remind people that vintage clothing is cut smaller than modern clothing, so if you wear a medium in a new shirt, you should probably buy a large in a vintage one. So when this guy accused me of deceptive marketing and called me all kinds of names, I was really upset.

When something like this happens, mindfulness tells me to take a deep breath and c-a-l-m d-o-w-n so I can think rationally and tell myself, *I don't have to react blindly to this; I can take a moment and make a reasonable response.* My heart rate goes down, my blood pressure subsides, my mind returns to the moment, and I can write a reasonable email to my customer.

I dedicate time to mindfulness every day. My living room has tall windows that look out on Little Cottonwood Canyon, where the bases of two mountains form a V. Mountains make me feel humble; they signify timelessness and remind me that they will endure long after I'm gone, which is comforting to me. I like to sit on my couch and gaze out at the mountains.

If it's nighttime or if I'm practicing mindfulness away from home, I close my eyes and picture them in my mind. I start by inhaling through my nose, filling my lungs with air, and exhaling through my mouth. I count to five during each step—inhaling, holding, then exhaling—to slow my breathing and focus on what is happening. All the while, I am mindful of the breath coming into my nose, then filling my lungs, and exiting through my mouth. I do this every day, ideally for fifteen minutes. Sometimes it's only for three, but I try to do it every day. It's a practice, which means I'll never master it, but I don't have to. It doesn't require a mat or incense or tea or a special room. All it requires is for me to still my body and focus my mind.

2 Higher Power

The most important aspect of the higher power concept is that you've got to be all in. There are no half measures. In its early days, AA had a distinctly Christian feel. The third step still urges participants to turn their lives over to God as they understand Him. But things have changed at AA, which now acknowledges that not all people are comfortable with the Christian concept of God, or any concept, for that matter. That's why we're now encouraged to identify our own higher power when we join a Twelve Step program.

My first week in rehab, an older gentleman explained that a higher power didn't have to be God; just believe in something that is greater than yourself and which could restore you to sanity. It could be the mountains, the ocean, or a tree. One teenager chose a dragonfly, although I cannot imagine an insect restoring me to sanity; usually, it's the other way around. For me, the choice was easy. God is my higher power, and I understand Him to be all that I need to get through life in this world.

When I was drinking, vodka was my higher power, and my life spun out of control. I was completely unable to manage my impulses, myself, my life. That is why I am more than happy to turn my life over to God, who I believe has a plan for me. All I have to do is to lay my worries to Him. Before, when I became worried about something, I'd freak out, lose control, and reach for a bottle to numb the chaos in my mind. Now when I start to worry, I remind myself that all I have to do is focus on this moment, this event, this day, and my higher power will take care of everything else.

But that's me, not you. You get to choose your higher power. The Twelve Traditions has been adapted to many different faith groups, cultures, and countries. There's a book by a rabbi and a doctor outlining a Jewish approach to the Twelve Steps, and another by an American Indian organization that adapts the Steps for Native Americans. A friend of mine was attending a book launch in Cadiz, Spain, and saw a poster advertising a meeting of *Alcohólicos Anónimos: UniTom, Servicio, Recuperacion*—unity, service, recovery. The language is different but the message is the same. Choose whomever or whatever you please. It can be anyone or anything. It doesn't matter, as long as you believe that it is greater and more powerful than you.

Rx

I was struggling with my back at the end of my time at Cirque Lodge. It was getting very painful to walk and be present in process groups. On May 2, 2012, I graduated and moved to Mom's house as a sort of sober living and recovery support. I also needed a third back surgery which I had in June. I thought it was going to fix all of my problems as that is what the surgeon assured me, but after a few weeks my back and sciatic nerve pain was worse than ever.

This surgeon botched my surgery, and I was devastated. The surgeries took so much out of me. I was hoping to have a healthy back again, but in fact, I was broken even more. I tried everything from epidural shots in my spine with steroids to bring the swelling down, to massive amounts of Tylenol and maxing out my post-surgery pain medications. But in the end, I was bedridden and almost out of hope.

One morning, I called a few doctors inquiring about performing a drop-leg procedure. No one would consider doing it until one eventually said he would, but strongly advised me against it.

When I asked why, he firmly said, "Mr. Kruse, once I cut your sciatica nerve, it will never grow back. You will no longer have any feeling in your left leg, but you will also not know you've broke the ankle until you smell it because you won't feel it."

That scared me enough to pursue another surgery, but this time it was done in Utah by a world-renowned orthopedic surgeon, Dr. K. My fourth surgery was finally a success. It was July 2013.

After the surgeon completed the fusion of my L5 S1 discs, I was lying in bed recovering. My doctor came in to check on me and reminded me to not make any sudden moves for the first 48 hours as my back needed to really accept the new bolts and screws he placed in me.

After he left, my mom was sitting next to me making sure I was good when the nurse came in to give me some medicine. I was groggy and reached around the table directly over me to accept the meds from her. She leaned on the table, which was on wheels, and in a blink of an eye she slipped forward and promptly braced her hand for balance right on the catheter that was attached to my penis!

I jumped straight up and yelled in pain, then remembered I wasn't supposed to make any sudden moves. The nurse was so embarrassed; she profusely apologized but when Mom saw this, she jumped up screaming in horror. A

practically overwhelming cacophony ensued, complete calamity with screaming and moaning! I thought to myself,
here I had waited months to get this massive surgery and
now it was ruined.

The nurse went running out the room; Mom was sobbing,
and all I could think about were the bolts I just popped out of
my freshly cut back. By the grace of God nothing happened,
and I healed after eight weeks. After this procedure, I have
since been pain-free. God blessed me with this alternative
surgery, and I regained my life. Hope got me there; I may
never have been able to walk again. Now I can walk my favorite trails in Utah, I can run with my daughter, and camp with
Lizzy. It's been a pure blessing and miracle, and the message
is to *never give up hope!*

3 Do What's Best for YOU: Self-Love is the Best Love

Put yourself first, because when you do what's best for you,
it works out better for everyone else too. It's not about ignoring
others' needs, but about weighing your needs against the needs
of others and giving yourself a fair shake. Many of us have been
trained to believe that putting ourselves last is a virtue, and in
some cases, it is. But when you habitually relegate your needs
to second, third, or last place, you're doing a disservice to both
yourself and the people you love.

I need my coffee in the morning. I have a busy schedule with
my self-employment, a wife and a child to support, and all of the
responsibilities that just come with living. I also know that my
mood and physical competence are dependent on ingesting some
caffeine. This is one very minor way in which I put myself first.

My personal appearance is another example. Some people used to let me know that they weren't crazy about my sobriety beard, especially when it became very long. They'd ask me why I was still growing it, or tell me how much better I'd look if I got rid of it. That's fine; they're entitled to their opinion. But growing that beard had meaning for me. I grew it not because of how it looked, but because it was a manifestation of how long I'd been sober. So I wasn't about to lose it because of how anyone else perceived it. Growing that beard was what was best for me, just as it was best for me to shave it off six years later.

If I show up for myself and do my best for myself, then I can show up for others and come through for them too. That's the biggest gift I or anyone else can give to others: to be fully present and fully engaged.

My mom has an affirmation: "If I do what's best for me today, it will be best for everyone I love in the long run." I'm with her one hundred percent. It takes different forms with different people. When I engage with a customer, it's different from the way I engage with my mom or with a friend. But if I take care of my own needs, I'm better able to tend to the needs of others, whether it's someone I work with or someone I love, like my daughter. It all starts with me . . . and, of course with my coffee.

Physical Integrity

By physical integrity I mean the maintenance of the body. My lack of it nearly did me in. I didn't go to the dentist for nineteen years; I'm lucky my teeth didn't fall out (I did have to pay over a thousand dollars to deal with the damage, some of which is irreversible). When you're young, you take your body for granted and assume it will always be hearty and strong. You don't realize that your body is a reflection of your self-respect, and the way you treat it reveals just how much, or how little, you esteem yourself.

In my using years, I didn't care how I treated my body or what I put into it. Oceans of alcohol, torrents of smoke, gobs of sugar, salt, and fat; I lived in an orgy of sensation and didn't give a damn about the body God had given me and what I owed it. Nor did I understand that it was the only body I was going to get, and if I didn't take care of it, it wouldn't take care of me.

Living in Recovery is a long-term commitment, a way of life. It's an acknowledgment that you did things in the past that compromised your future health, and now it's your responsibility to repair what you broke. Exercising is part of it and so is eating healthy food. But another part of it is changing the way you think about your body, and learning to honor it for the miracle that it is.

After all my back surgeries, the reason I am still pain free is my maintenance program. A minimum of three times a week, two-and-a-half miles at a time, like it or not, rain, snow, or shine, I walk briskly to get my heart rate up and keep it up. I don't find excuses to not do my walk because I don't ever want to endure that agony again. When the surgeon discharged me and told me I had to walk, I took it seriously. Not only did it help me recover from the surgery; every time I do it, I feel that I am honoring my body and doing it a service.

5 Emotional Ownership, or See a Therapist

I was an emotional kid, and I'm an emotional man. It's ironic that my emotions are God-given gifts, yet I spent so many years numbing myself so I wouldn't feel them. One of the blessings of sobriety is having the stability and strength to acknowledge my emotions and feel them fully, knowing that their purpose is to give me information about my psychological well-being, just as my senses provide information about the well-being of my body.

I experienced therapy for the first time when I went into rehab, and I cannot express how much it has helped me. Therapy gave me techniques for managing emotions that used to overwhelm me, like when Tom tricked me into carrying that obscene photo to my mom.

I was so furious, I burned up the highway all the way home, screaming, "What the hell just happened?" in the car. I was so angry, so hurt, so sad, so jacked up by all the feelings, the only way I could survive them was to drink myself into a stupor when I got home. I didn't know how to experience the feelings and deal with them. The only thing I knew to do was to obliterate them, and in the process, myself.

When I stopped drinking, I became anxious in ways I'd never been before. This was when I began experiencing my problems driving on the highway; every time I got behind the wheel, I would see a big movie screen filled with images of the death and destruction that were going to happen to me. This was still happening well after rehab, when my back was healed, and I was living in Utah, where you need to use the highway to get places.

My therapist said there was a cognitive-behavioral therapy technique he wanted me to try. "The next time you're driving, shrink that movie screen down from your windshield-size to a tiny TV screen sitting on the dashboard. Then reach over and put it on the passenger seat and tell it, 'I know you're there and I know my brain is trying to keep me safe. But the catastrophe I fear that is going to happen will only be on your little screen; I'm going to look through my windshield and not watch you.'

I do that to this day, especially in heavy traffic when cars are darting around me, and I start to feel antsy and imagine what could happen. I just shrink the images down to that tiny square, use my fingers like tweezers to put it down out of my line of sight and say, "You're right there." It works every time.

Another thing I do is take a low daily dose of an anti-depressant. It's a selective serotonin re-uptake inhibitor (SSRI), which means it regulates the brain's transmission of chemicals, which can mitigate anxiety as well as depression. It is a non-narcotic and is not habit-forming. It just takes what my body is producing too much of and brings it down to a normal level.

Living in Recovery means honoring my feelings and acknowledging that they are real. If I'm really sad, I give myself permission to cry. If I'm really angry, I scream and yell (preferably by myself behind a closed door). If I'm confused, I search out an answer. Whatever I'm feeling, I honor it by letting it go through my body. Then I release it.

6 Play the Tape Through

I learned this technique in rehab, and it's a big arrow in the quiver of Recovery. The tape refers to a video tape on which is recorded what would likely happen if you satisfied your urge to use your drug of choice. The technique suggests you play the tape through to the end to remind yourself of the consequences of relapsing.

Imagine I'm driving past a bar where I used to get wasted. If I go in and buy a drink, I break my sobriety. What would I do next? I'd hate myself for doing that, so I'd buy a bottle of vodka and drink all night. Next, I'd go to work drunk the next day and not get my orders out. Next, I'd go out and drown my sorrows in more vodka. Next, I'd get behind the wheel and either cause an accident and damage my car, cause an accident and damage someone else's car, injure myself or someone else, or even kill myself or someone else.

That's playing the tape through: looking at what might happen if I did this one risky thing and asking myself, *Is it worth it? You're about to screw up your life again, Nate. Is it worth it? No!*

The longer you're sober, the more you have to lose. Playing the tape through forces you to slow down, think, and take stock of your options. It defuses the power of the trigger. It puts you back in control.

7 Fear: Forget Everything and Run, or Face Everything and Recover

I love this root. When I first learned it, the *forget every-thing* part used a different *F* word, and still does in Recovery circles. I'll mostly stick with *forget* here, but you're welcome to *F* everything in your head (I still do).

This one clicked for me right away. It's one of my biggest motivators, because if I'm afraid of something, I'm not going to do it. The way I ignored my two DUIs is a perfect example. I was so afraid of doing time, a warrant was issued for my arrest. I was so afraid of getting arrested, I ruined my life for nineteen years. Fear held me back in so many ways.

When I had a mountain of debt, I said *"F" it!* and ran. When I was dating a woman and things got serious, my emotional immaturity and lack of confidence would say, *F it, man! Run!* And that's what I did. I'd feel free in the moment, imagining I'd cut myself loose from the commitment I was so afraid of. But after a few days I would miss the companionship and feel terrible.

Now I face everything: bills, disputes with customers, disagreements with family; I even faced my DUIs.

8 Under-Commit and Over-Deliver

This root is not about doing less than you're able to; it's knowing what you're capable of, living up to that standard, and exceeding it whenever possible. It's being choosy about what you'll commit to, and, if you commit, doing your best to fulfill the commitment. It's not overselling yourself to make a good impression, an easy sale, or a quick buck. It's exercising your powers of discretion so that when you do commit, you know you can come through. This principle has worked in my professional life and in my personal life. If I say I'm going to do something, I do it.

The only way I can differentiate myself on *EBay* is to maintain a one hundred percent satisfaction score, and I do. If I say I'm going to ship an order within forty-eight hours of receiving payment, I'd better do that. It doesn't matter if there's a hurricane, tornado, or whatever: that order had better be in the mail within forty-eight hours. And if I'm not able to ship an order on time, I'd better have a good reason (such as when my daughter was born) and contact my customers to tell them that there's going to be a holdup. That's how I under-commit: I know that forty-eight hours is more than enough time for me to ship an order. Ninety-five percent of the time, I ship in less than twenty-four hours, and that's how I over-deliver: my customers almost always get their orders sooner than they expected.

It comes down to being honest with other people as well as myself. I don't commit to a twenty-four-hour turnaround because sometimes there are delays I can't control, and it wouldn't be forthright to pretend otherwise. Being honest implies I respect the person I'm in a relationship with, whether personal or professional. I can't even count the number of people I've met who swear they're going to do something, then don't do it, and don't tell me.

I used to be notorious for doing just that. I once made plans to go golfing with a friend, and we arranged to meet outside at seven on Saturday morning. I partied all night Friday, passed out on my mattress, and woke up to find him standing over me in my bedroom in a pristine golf polo, shouting, "Nate, it's seven o'clock! We've got to be on the green in twenty minutes!" I could not move: my head was throbbing and my limbs wouldn't work. I said, "Sorry, man, I totally forgot." He was angry; it wasn't the first time I'd done this. I felt guilty for letting him down yet again. I had over-committed and under-delivered. The other way around is better.

9 Have No Expectations

I also think of this root as the "We'll see" approach, because it increases the odds that I'll be grateful for the outcome, whatever it is.

Having no expectations, or at least low ones, is vital to Recovery. If you expect things to turn out a certain way and they fall short, you're going to be disappointed. Disappointment breeds resentment and resentment is toxic, because it feels terrible and makes you want to lose yourself in your drug of choice.

When I went into rehab, my expectation was that in my first year of sobriety, I would be healed of alcoholism, get a good job, meet a nice woman, and get back with my old friends. Instead, decades of buried emotions started to surface. I was stricken with anxiety, and I thought, *Wait—this is bullshit! This isn't what I signed up for; it's supposed to be easier, not harder!* I began to question why I thought I had the guts to get sober. *What had I gotten myself into? Was it even worth it?* I'd sworn off alcohol, but I still wanted to drink; I was crippled with a bad back and couldn't work; I didn't have a girlfriend, and I felt disconnected from my old drinking friends. That was hard. It would have been hard in any case, but what made it much harder were my unrealistic expectations.

If I could do it over again, I would approach sobriety thinking "We'll see" instead of expecting to check off every box on my to-do list. I'd think, *Let me take just the first task and do the best I can, see what happens, and take it from there.* It's a close relative of under-committing and over-delivering, focused on you rather than others. This root requires you to under-commit and over-deliver to *yourself*. It feels bad to disappoint others, but it can feel worse to disappoint yourself. Lowering your expectations makes it more likely that you'll meet them and even exceed them.

10 Surround Yourself with Like-Minded People and Ask for Help When You Need It

I'm at the post office almost every day, and I've become friendly with a woman who works there. She always has a smile on her face and that smile lifts me up. I feel her vibration, and my soul is happy when it meets her soul. I walk out of there feeling better than when I walked in, and that boosts the odds that I'll have a decent day. That feeling of uplift, of connecting with a joyful human spirit, is at the center of this root and also the success of AA.

At an AA meeting, you're surrounded by people fighting the same demons you are. Not everyone is upbeat; some people are struggling. But there's an atmosphere of optimism and faith that things can and will get better. I know I cannot do Recovery alone. I know I need other people. And when I need help, I ask for it.

It's not always easy to admit I need help. Early in my sobriety, I accompanied my mom to a party in Idaho hosted by her friend John Southworth, now deceased, who was active in the Recovery movement. This was when I was struggling with intense anxiety and hadn't yet dealt with it in therapy. I hadn't dealt with it at all, in fact, because I felt ashamed. I had this idea that I should be able to fix it myself. I know better now, but at the time it was hard for me to admit I couldn't just get a grip on myself and make the problem go away. So the next morning at breakfast, I took a deep breath and told my mom that I was barely functioning because I was having panic attacks.

"Oh, Nate," she said, "you can't just stop panic attacks from happening. It's not your fault." She said she'd talk to a woman she knew who'd attended the party with her husband, who happened to be a psychiatrist. And an hour later, I was sitting in his hotel room, telling him what I was going through and asking if there was anything that could be done about it. He said yes, there was, and that he thought a low dose of an antidepressant might do the trick. I went to see my doctor when I got home, and that's when I began taking a daily dose of Paxil. That, and the miniature TV technique my therapist taught me, gave me back my freedom.

Ever since then, when I need help, I ask for it. That's why I surround myself with like-minded people, so when I approach them with a problem, they sincerely want to help. Now that I'm in Recovery, I cannot afford to put my faith in untrustworthy people. I know I can't control what other people say and do, but I can control who my friends are. Choosing positive, optimistic people to hang out with boosts the odds that I'll maintain my sobriety over the long haul.

11 Be a Lion, Not a Sheep

This root is about breaking the mold that your parents, your family, your friends, or your culture is trying to fit you into. It encourages you to roar, not bleat; assert, not recede; manifest, not disappear. It urges you to be your own leader and not follow the path that society prescribes for you. *Society is other people.* They don't know you as well as you do, so they can't know what's best for you.

In the old days, when people asked me what I did for a living and I said I sold insurance, they'd say, "Wow, that's great!" I knew better; I knew I was miserable and lost and hated the work, but "insurance salesman" labeled me as a solid, solvent citizen, even though I was anything but.

Now when I tell people about my business, they say, "Wow! Can you really make a living doing that?" I tell them not only do I make a living, I love every minute of it. It was the lion in me that told me I could make a career out of this, that I should harness my passion for finding things and ride it into a new way of living.

I now see it was the sheep in me that kept trusting Tom when, deep down, I knew I shouldn't. He taught me never to question him, that he ruled the family, and his word was law. Even when the evidence proved that his word was dirt, I refused to take it in, preferring to follow the edicts of my culture and society: *He's your dad. He's your blood. Family comes first. A good son trusts his father.* No: an oblivious son trusts his father when the father has proved he cannot be trusted. The day I stopped calling him Dad was the day a lion cub was born in me.

When I was growing up, most people thought an addict or alcoholic was a dirty guy in ragged clothes, with run-down shoes and stringy hair, pacing the street with a cigarette dangling from his mouth. Things have gotten a little better, but we're not there yet: people with addictions are still stigmatized. Some people still believe that if I'm an alcoholic in Recovery, it means I'm a deviant, a self-indulgent person with no self-control. They don't see me as a person with a disease, but as a weakling who can't manage his out-sized appetites. That's why I understand why some people hide the fact that they're in Recovery. To me, it's a personal choice. No one is morally obliged to reveal that they weren't always sober. But for me, being a lion means being forthright about who I am and what I've been through. If I'm hiding who I am, I'll never be my true self.

12 Sobriety Means Taking Responsibility

I sometimes describe this root as "Pull the thumb; don't point the finger." It comes from the image of pointing your finger at someone as if you're accusing them. The idea is to pull back on your thumb until it touches your chest—your heart—rather than pointing your finger and blaming someone else. To me, it's a visualization of accountability, of examining my own motives and actions before judging those of other people.

This one took me a while to digest and put into effect. I had made so many excuses for so long, I'd convinced myself that I was a victim of the universe's ill-will. I understand now that I was a victim when I was little, mostly because of the examples of bad behavior of adults surrounding me. But as a sober adult, I understand that no one owes me anything. To succeed at Recovery long term, I need to take responsibility for everything I say and do.

If I'm on a long phone call with someone and become testy because I haven't eaten all day, it's my responsibility to tell them I'm hungry and will call back after I have something to eat. My DUIs are another example. When I moved back to Jacksonville, I couldn't get a Florida license because the DUIs would pop up, and I'd be nailed.

I carried on about it for years, blaming it on the Scottsdale cops who pulled me over. I was pointing the finger at them when I should have pulled the thumb back at myself. The arrest warrant was my fault, not theirs.

A good way to live this root is to practice making "I" statements rather than "you" statements, as in, "I get anxious when the door isn't locked at night," rather than, "You forgot to lock the door again!" This way, I get my point across without blaming someone else for falling short. I've made my point by speaking only of myself, and the other person doesn't feel triggered into defensiveness.

10 Give Back, Donate Your Time, Be Kind

There's a saying in the Recovery movement that goes, "The only way to keep your sobriety is to give it away." That's the soul of this root, that by giving of myself, investing time in others, and treating them with kindness, I encourage their sobriety while strengthening my own.

Living this root takes a variety of forms. It means showing up with a positive attitude every day, no matter what problems I'm dealing with. It means paying attention and opening a door for someone pushing a stroller, woman or man, or offering to help someone put groceries in a car. It means making eye contact with people when they talk to me, and resisting the temptation to blast the horn when the driver in front of me is too slow for my taste.

I share a lot about my Recovery on social media. Someone I knew in high school reached out to me on Facebook; she wanted to talk about her sister, whose alcohol and drug use had dangerously escalated since their mother died a few years earlier. She said that reading about my recovery gave her hope for her sister and she asked for advice. I was honored to know this, and I told her what I had done to get sober. This is the ultimate compliment, that my actions spark hope in people who are struggling.

You can show kindness and caring in any setting as long as you have the courage to tell the truth and share your victories. This past year, I became a certified peer support specialist, which means I've been trained to provide empathy and encouragement to people in Recovery. Talking to newly sober men and women, meeting with them and cheering them on, is deeply rewarding for me. It gives meaning to all the years I was floundering and lost. That's giving back: telling others who need to hear, "What happened to you, happened to me. I rose above it, and so can you."

14 You Can't Heal in the Place Where You got Sick

In rehab, they made a point of telling me that when I returned home to Jacksonville, I'd be right back where I got sick and did bad things to myself. "You don't have to live there," my therapist said. "You can live somewhere else and give yourself a fresh start."

This had never occurred to me. In my mind, Jacksonville was the only place I could live: my brother and his family were there, my friends were there; it was my home. Then I left Cirque early for Mississippi to have back surgery. Lying in my mom's house in pain for four months, I had time to contemplate what to do next. You've been sober for 210 days, I told myself. Why would you go back to a place where all you did was drink? Everything in Jacksonville reminded me of drinking, and still does. I actually get triggered when the city pops up on TV. When the Jaguars play on ESPN and I'm watching, I'm transported back to the scene of the crime.

There's a certain smell in Jacksonville when the sun goes down, a humid, grassy aroma that reminded me that it was time to knock off work, light a cigarette, and down some vodka. I knew myself well enough to know that I'd have to overcome tremendous obstacles to maintain my sobriety there. That knowledge, as well as learning that Utah had both low humidity and lots of surgeons who might be able to fix my back, persuaded me to move West. If I was going to stay sober, I had to set myself up for success and start my new phase of life in a new place.

This decision should not be confused with what's known as a geographical fix: the idea that your problems don't originate in yourself but in your surroundings, and that if you pack up and move somewhere else, your problems will vanish. It doesn't work, of course: we take our problems with us wherever we go. All the places my parents moved—from Nebraska to Illinois to Michigan to Nebraska to Kansas to California to Germany to Florida to Arizona—if relocating could fix people's problems, we'd have been the happy family we were pretending to be. But nothing gets better until you address the root of the problem. For my mom, it meant removing her drug of choice, which was Tom. For me, it meant removing alcohol, which was mine.

The essence of this root is simple: sometimes you have to leave home to come home to your true self.

15 Acceptance

This root is hard to put into practice. A passage in *The Big Book* (p. 417) describes it better than I can:

"When I am disturbed, it is because I find some person, place, thing, or situation—some fact of my life—unacceptable to me, and I can find no serenity until I accept that person, place, thing, or situation as being exactly the way it is supposed to be at this moment. Nothing, absolutely nothing, happens in God's world by mistake. Until I could accept my alcoholism, I could not stay sober; unless I accept life completely on life's terms, I cannot be happy. I need to concentrate not so much on what needs to be changed in the world as on what needs to be changed in me and in my attitudes."

RX

Learning to accept the world as it is—not as I would like it to be—is a cornerstone of my Recovery. In rehab, as I was dealing with the wreckage of my past and the anxiety of facing the future, the winds of my life were blowing very hard, and the concept of acceptance was an anchor, keeping me fixed in my harbor of sobriety. It's the heart of the serenity prayer, in which we ask for the wisdom to recognize when we can't change something and to accept its existence whether we like it or not. As frustrating as it feels at first, it's actually a form of liberation, because it frees us from the obligation to engage in a struggle that is ultimately hopeless.

This is not just a Recovery issue; *it's a life issue.* All around me—literally—are things that drive me nuts. The car in front of me who's doing twenty-five in a forty-five mile per hour zone; the person behind me talking so loudly on her phone that I can't hear my own thoughts; the friend who makes plans only to cancel with a lame excuse at the last minute (just as I used to do); the people I love whose habits are different from mine; the institutions whose rules and regulations seem designed to thwart my efforts to right my wrongs. That is exactly what happened when I made the decision to finally deal with my DUIs and the arrest warrant. So many officials pushed obstacles into my path, I was in despair that I'd ever be able to make things right.

My therapist sat me down and said, "Whatever you do, don't give up. You must accept this the way it is. This is how they do things here and you can't change it. We'll figure out later why it happened this way. But now, you must accept." I felt so much animosity that if I hadn't been forced to accept things as they were, I would have started to drink again to dull the frustration. I was at my breaking point when I received the wisdom that I must accept life on its terms, not mine.

Bill W. said, "We didn't get sober just to go to meetings." He was right. We get sober to live with other people in love, joy, and healing. Learning to accept those people in all their humanity is something I work on every day.

16 Get Shit Done

This root is about action. It reminds me to stop procrastinating and get done what I need to do. As a part-time stay-at-home dad, my to-do list is long. Between home chores and business chores, not to mention caring for my daughter, it would be easy to feel daunted. And sometimes I do: If I inundate myself with a long list of tasks, all I see is a deluge of obligations that I can't hope to fulfill. But by keeping it simple, doing one thing at a time and doing that one thing right, I'm able to accomplish a lot more than I thought I could.

Not long ago, my business had a windfall: twenty-three orders came in within twenty-four hours. I was ecstatic. I was also up with the baby all night, and when the sun rose, so did my anxiety level. How in the world would I package twenty-three orders, create mailing labels, and get them all to the post office before five o'clock, and, *oh yeah,* also take care of the baby, when I could barely focus my eyes?

I thought, *One thing at a time. What comes first?* That was easy: sleep. So when Josie dozed off after her bottle, I did too (no bottle for me). We slept for two hours, which wasn't as much as I needed but enough for me to function.

Okay, what next? I packed the diaper bag, put Josie in her car seat, and we headed off to my office, where I spent the morning preparing orders for shipment, napping with Josie after her lunchtime bottle, and preparing more orders that afternoon. I got nineteen out of twenty-three packed and out the door that day, and dispatched the remaining four the next morning, well within my forty-eight hour commitment. By deconstructing my mountain of obligations into small, manageable pieces, the seemingly impossible became manageable.

It's the same with Recovery: I can't imagine promising to never have another drink; even though it's my dream to stay sober, it's too vast a commitment for me to contemplate. Instead, I tell myself that I will not drink today. That is a promise I can keep. Splitting a big dream into smaller ones makes them attainable. Attaining even a small dream is a big deal.

17 Own and Cultivate Your Power

This root reminds me that I do have control; I do have power. The power I have is limited to myself, but that's all the power I need. If I exercise my personal power to manage myself—the way I approach my loved ones, my friends, my colleagues, my neighbors, my customers, my commitments, and my relationships with my fellow creatures—I am doing everything I morally and ethically can to live honorably.

The root of owning and cultivating your power has its own roots in the second step of Dr. Bob's prescription for sobriety: clean house. That's a metaphor for venturing into every room inside myself, facing what I find there, and cleaning up the wreckage of my past. That's where my power lies: in cleaning my inner house, the place my mom calls the home of the self. I'm the only one who can do it, and when I don't, it becomes cluttered with unfinished emotional business that prevents me from knowing my feelings and acting in appropriate ways.

It wasn't until rehab that I took ownership of this power, because I never knew I had it. The great shift that happened was recognizing that I am worth all the hard work it takes to live a sober life. I am worthy of this journey. When I was drinking, I saw myself as the victim of fate and other people's willfulness. There was just enough truth in that perception to perpetuate it. People are going to do what they do; we cannot control them. But what I didn't see and couldn't own was my capacity to respond mindfully rather than react mindlessly. That's the essence of cleaning house, of cleaning my side of the street.

This has included making a list of people I may have wronged, and then visiting those people, face to face, and saying, "I may have hurt you during my active alcoholism, and if I did, please tell me how I can make amends." This is step number eight of the twelve: to face the people you have either wronged or believe you may have wronged, and ask how you can make it up to them. It heals my soul to make things right. That's how to cultivate your power: by making amends. To build my power from within, I have to own that I have been unkind and admit that I'm wrong. When I was drinking, I could never admit I was wrong. Now I can, and I do.

When I did the Ring of Fire at Cirque with Mom and we pictured Tom in a chair and howled our pain over all he'd done to us, then took that chair outside and smashed it to smithereens, *I gained back my power.* I could feel it in my body, as if a straitjacket of rage was untied and lifted off me. Part of it was the physical exertion of exorcising the fury I'd been harboring for so long. The other part was what my therapist said: "You must forgive the people who hurt you. Don't do it for them; do it for yourself." I don't think I could ever forgive Tom to his face, but I could forgive him for my own sake, for my own peace of heart and mind. Purging rage through forgiveness is another way of cleaning house.

I couldn't see it at the time, but when our neighbors threw broken glass in front of our home in Germany, and we went outside to sweep it up, we were acting out a metaphor. We were cleaning our side of the street. The emotional burdens others heap upon us are like those broken bottles. We may not have put them there, but it's still up to us to get rid of them. It's useless to rant against the injustice of it all. All we can do is face the wreckage, pick up a broom, and get to work.

18 Celebrate Victories

This root is another nugget of wisdom from my therapist, who left Cirque after I did to go into private practice, and who I continued to see occasionally for maintenance therapy. I'd been sober for about two years when he asked me during a session if I was taking the time to celebrate all I'd accomplished. I told him *no, I wasn't.* I just did what I did and kept on going. "Look," he said, "recovery has no finish line; you're never going to cross a threshold and get a trophy. There is no end to recovery, which is why you must celebrate every victory as it happens. If you don't, you'll never realize how far you've come." I saw his point. We call it a journey, but it's a journey without end. We're never going to have a ta-da! moment with one big triumph. Our triumphs are usually small and come without fanfare: declining a sip of Champagne at a wedding; forgoing guys' night out at a bar; passing on a trip to Vegas. They're invisible except to us, and that's why we should celebrate them, because no one else will. And those hidden, seemingly invisible experiences that still plague us subconsciously? Well, they need to be addressed eventually too.

It was April 2018, and Lizzy just discovered she was pregnant. I was ecstatic, but at the same time, I knew it was time to reveal the "plague" that had been following me for years. I could not bring a child into our world with this hanging over my head. It was a danger to me, to Lizzy, and to this new life to come.

So, I told Lizzy that I had a second DUI from when I lived in Arizona that I had run from, and it may mean I would have to spend some time in jail. I was certain that the hammer would fall, and she would crush me with this revelation. But no; not my Lizzy. I could not believe that she could be so positive and so accepting, actually supporting me on this journey to clear up the final piece of my past wreckage!

We were on a beautiful hike one day in Sundance after visiting Cirque and telling them the news of our pregnancy. Lizzy and I were deep in the mountains and came across a piece of bone. It looked like a pelvic bone from a small animal. It clicked in my head, and I made the connection that this bone represented the final skeleton in my closet that held me back for almost 17 years.

I picked up the bone and felt God's power again. He was showing me that this was it, this was the time to make good with my past, do the hard work and trust Him that it would all work out. I was six years sober and felt very secure in my Recovery. I had the tools to get through this and be free for myself and my family. I had the help of my amazing therapist who really guided my emotions and kept feeding me positivity as things became hard.

So in the end, I have faced my biggest fear and given my pound of flesh to the great state of Arizona; and I'm now free. I will always have that piece of bone. It sits in my office as a reminder that I have the strength to face and conquer anything in my life.

RX

I'm involved with Cirque outreach programs, one of which is a virtual process group that meets digitally for conversations about Recovery. We had one a while back that included a new resident, a woman in her late twenties who had been addicted to crystal meth. She couldn't bring herself to look at the camera, and, staring down at her lap, said that when she was admitted to Cirque, it was the first time in six years that she had brushed her teeth twice every day for a week straight. "It made me feel human again," she said, and began to cry. My heart lurched: Who would think that brushing your teeth would feel like a victory? But for this woman, it was an act of self-love, a manifestation of a self-respect she had not felt in years. I congratulated her on her victory and said that every time she picked up her toothbrush was another victory too.

My DUI demons are dead. Dealing with them is one of the victories I celebrate every day. It's the next and final story I have to tell.

*Set your heart
on doing good.
Do it over and over again and
you
will be filled with joy.*
—Buddha

POSTSCRIPT

Surrender. People say your life changes forever when you have a child. Mine changed sooner. The moment I learned I was going to be a father, I knew the jig was up. Next to getting sober, this was the biggest thing that had ever happened, would ever happen, could ever happen to me. In nine months, a brand new person, *my child* would arrive in the world and look to me for comfort, care, and love. I wanted this child to know me and trust me. For that to happen, I had to come clean.

My parents knew about my first DUI. I didn't advertise the second, although Tom and my brother may have known about it when I got back to Florida. But no one knew I hadn't handled it. No one knew I was supposed to do jail time and never did. No one knew there was a warrant out for my arrest. For seventeen years, the secret had eaten away at my self-respect and peace of mind. I lived in dread of attracting the attention of a cop. I was haunted by the threat of being apprehended, handcuffed, and thrown into jail.

I decided to take charge and turn myself in. I would not wait to be caught. Even if the very worst were to occur—jail—I would surrender. There is power in surrendering, in agreeing to yield control to someone else. I had a choice and I would make it: that was one thing I could control. The skeleton in my closet had rattled me long enough. I was ready to yank it into the light and see what it, *and I,* were made of.

I searched Arizona's government websites. I made phone calls. I wrote emails. I found out what I needed to do to clear my record. I learned that some states, in some cases, permitted people to serve time under ankle monitoring surveillance rather than in a brick-and-mortar jail. I found out that the Salt Lake City Police Department used ankle monitoring but had never approved it for someone who was wanted in another state. I decided to find out if they'd make an exception for me. I made more phone calls and wrote more emails. I cited my stint in rehab, six years of sobriety, and a thriving business, which I might lose if I went to jail. I wrote letters and faxed records and documents. When I became discouraged by the bureaucratic gobbledygook and enraged by the runarounds, my therapist counseled me to stop fighting the system, accept it, keep on going, and get shit done.

It paid off. I got approved for ankle monitoring. I felt elation, triumph, vindication, trepidation. But most of all, I felt hope.

I drove to Salt Lake City and surrendered myself to the County Sheriff's Department on a warm May morning. They were waiting for me because I was the first person ever to serve time at a Salt Lake jail for an out-of-state offense and there was no protocol for how to process me. This ended up being a miracle because a deputy stayed with me the whole time and walked me through.

I was handcuffed and taken down a flight of stairs to a lower level where the deputy banged loudly on a metal door. The door clanged and slid open, and I was led to a concrete slab that passed for a bench with a metal rail onto which they fastened my cuffs. The deputy said to sit, wait, be cool, do what they tell you, and keep your mouth shut. I thought, *Amen, brother, whatever you say.* I sat and waited. My nerves were jangling, adrenaline flowing. Every sense was humming. Sounds were louder, sights were more vivid. I never realized how cold concrete could be.

A guard came, detached me from the slab, and told me to undress: shoes, socks, shirt, pants, everything came off except my underwear. I was told to face the wall and put my hands up against it, and spread my feet while I got frisked and they went through all the pockets in my clothes. "You're good," he said, "get dressed." I did. Then my deputy walked me to another metal door, which he banged on. It slid open and I was looking at "the pit," a huge space with a sunken floor in the center and raised banks of cops at desks on the right and holding cells on the left.

I saw where they got the name from. The sunken area was packed with maybe twenty men and women who had been arrested the night before. Some were drunk or strung out on drugs; others were slumped on benches or the floor, eyes glazed, glaring, or closed. More than a few were staring up at me. The place stunk of vomit, urine, and sweat. My deputy told me to keep quiet because if I said anything, they'd throw me in a cell. He wasn't kidding. The holding cells had doors that were metal on the bottom and Plexiglas on top, and I looked up and saw two people, high on drugs or drink, eyes wild, pounding on their doors and screaming.

This is where they processed people they'd arrested, and mercy found me again, because they fast-tracked me, and I wasn't sent down into the pit. A guard asked me, "You a celebrity or something?" I told him no; why did he ask? "See all those people down there? They've been waiting ten hours, some of them, to get processed, and you're skipping ahead of everyone." It was a miracle, and I knew it. They took a mug shot and my fingerprints, then sent me to an officer at a desk who asked me questions about who I was, where I lived, and the reason for my arrest. He asked for my driver's license and when I told him I didn't have one, he looked up.

"What are you talking about?" he asked. I told him it was suspended after two DUIs. "You've been driving for seventeen years on a suspended license?" he asked. "Yes," I said. I had. "Never been stopped by a cop?" No, never. He just shook his head.

My next destination was to see the discharge clerk who gave me my official intake papers, I was supplied with an ankle monitor and instructions as to how to use, where and what I could do, and Lizzy came and brought me home.

I was required to come to the Sheriff's Department every week for a urinalysis and meet with a deputy. The fourth week, my deputy said, "How long do you think you'll live in Utah?"

"I love it here," I said. "A long time."

"Did you used to smoke?"

"I sure did. Twenty years."

"Nate," he said, "your recovery is something that we rarely see; you're in the top one percent. We need to see more of your kind of success. We run this outreach program but so many people break the rules and get high, get drunk, get rearrested. People need to know how you do it, how you're managing to succeed."

He then told me that the state of Utah had just instituted a new program to train former addicts to work with people who were new to sobriety. After forty hours of training, graduates were certified to spend time, one-on-one, with people in recovery, not as therapists or coaches, but as survivors of addiction who wanted to help fellow travelers on their recovery journeys. They would listen, empathize, encourage, and, if appropriate, share information about what had worked for them. The prerequisite was that trainees had to have been sober for at least one year.

I signed up for the training, which I could start as soon as I'd finished serving my sentence. On July 23, 2018, my 41st birthday, my ankle monitor came off. Six months later, I graduated as a Peer Support Specialist, certified by the Utah Department of Human Services, Division of Substance Abuse and Mental Health. I could not believe my ears: this was my dream come true.

I have worked with about six people so far, some in person, some on the phone. A woman I went to high school with contacted me through social media. She's newly sober and struggling, so she calls me once a week to check in and tell me what she's facing. I listen, empathize, and suggest possible positive outcomes to what she perceives as purely negative situations.

Also, Cirque has called me to support some residents who have just gotten out of treatment. One of them, a married father in his thirties, was twenty-eight days sober when he texted and asked to meet for coffee. He said he was anxious about reentry into his old life and needed support. We sat for two hours while he asked what I went through and how I coped with early times in recovery. We discussed the potential issues he was facing, and I shared ways I had approached similar ones. We plan to meet again.

Peer support work nurtures my soul. It is my love and my passion to connect with other human beings and share my experience of self-destruction, the strength I've found in being sober, and the hope that, through my Recovery, I can share this gift that the Lord has blessed me with. It's an honor to have an impact on the lives of people who want to better themselves. Doing this work is the antithesis of who I was as an alcoholic. I was bankrupt emotionally, financially, spiritually, and physically. Now, my business has been up and running for seven years. I am finally in touch with who I truly am. And I have a better relationship with God than ever before.

God's not done with me yet, and neither is the Sheriff's Department. When the ankle monitor came off, a breathalyzer apparatus was installed in my car. It's hooked up to the ignition, and it won't let the car start until I prove I haven't been drinking. When I put in the key, I have to blow into a straw attached to the apparatus, and when it determines I'm alcohol-free, it sends a signal that allows the car to start. Not only that, ten minutes later, while I'm driving, the apparatus will beep and I have three minutes to blow again into the straw and take another test. If I wait longer than three minutes, the car will turn off, just like that, in the middle of the road. It was an inconvenience but it's a time-bound, fifteen-month automotive surveillance sentence that ended in the fall of 2019. By the time you read this, I will be apparatus-free, monitor-free, and warrant free.

Rx

Freedom has meant different things to me at different times. Now it means doing my best. I can't commit to doing a lot, but what I do commit to, I give it one hundred percent. Knowing I was going to be a father made me want to greet my child unfettered by secrecy, so I did my time, gave it my all, and freed myself from the past. Then, a few months before Josie was born, I felt a need to be known in a different way, and I shaved off my six-year-old sobriety beard so my child could know the real me and see my true face. That, too, felt like freedom.

By doing my best, I live miracles every day. It's a miracle that I was able to renounce the god of vodka and replace it with my true God, and a program so strong and so reliable that, whatever comes my way, I can take a deep breath, recite the serenity prayer, and respond rather than react. Doing my best means going all the way, no matter how tempting it is to quit, because Recovery is a marathon, not a sprint. It means looking at myself in the mirror and saying to the person looking back at me, "I am living this day for you. Whatever I do, I am going to do it one hundred percent."

RX

I remember times when I'd break down and cry, trying to let it out once in a while if I was with someone I trusted, but most of the time I acted like I was bulletproof. Nothing got to me. The more I drank the better I felt; the more I got high, the farther away I was from my family and the bad feelings.

It's different being sober. I still feel things all the time, including things I don't want to feel, but I have to feel in order to live. Anesthesia through drinking is no longer an option. You've probably heard that when someone's really drunk, they're feeling no pain? It's really just the opposite. When someone gets really drunk, it's because of the pain and getting drunk or high is the only way they can see to escape.

I continue to work at controlling my anger every day, so I get a lot of practice. But my child will never experience a childhood like mine because we'll do family vacations; create great memories, take lots of pictures, and come home and re-live the joy by going through those picture albums and recalling all the good times. For me, family time is what counts. The family is my glue that keeps joy inside and fear outside, for the most part. And it enables my partner and me to know what our child is experiencing so they will be less likely to fall into habits that could destroy them, and the family too.

I have built my life around the things that bring me joy and love. I live every day with an abundance of gratitude for the miracles and promises that have come true. Today, no amount of alcohol or drugs could match the enthusiasm I have for life and that is why I choose Recovery for these 24 hours. My life is so good, I don't want to mask it or alter it in any way.

It took 34 years and me going to rehab to understand this journey starts with me. A roommate of mine at Cirque, eight years ago, challenged me to look at my reflection in the mirror and say, "Nate, I love you." It was the first time in my life I did that, and it broke my heart to see the pain and damage I inflicted upon myself during my active addiction years.

I now embrace the moment and live life to the fullest, understanding it all starts and ends with me. I honor the fact that through my hard work and not giving up I am now worthy for these miracles, and I want to pass that feeling along to you, now. If you are deciding to start this journey of freedom through Recovery, then ask for help. We are out here for you.

If you are already on this journey, then don't give up. You and your story are needed to inspire the next person who needs your strength. We are all worthy because we are worth it. I will choose to take another 24 hours of being clean and living serene . . . will you join me?

*One moment
can change a day,
one day can
change a life,
and one life
can change the world.*

—Buddha

ACKNOWLEDGMENTS

This book has been a special journey for me, and I'm humbled to thank the following:

To my Mom: Thank you for answering your phone when I called at my worst moment. You are my hero and I respect and love you immensely. You were the catalyst for my recovery journey and I honor all that you have done for me.

To my beautiful Partner: Thank you for being everything, from reading early drafts, to giving me inspiration on the cover, to always being the best Mom for our daughter so I could write. You are as important to this book being completed as I was. You never gave up on me and pushed me to the highest level of success. We have dreamed big together and our dreams are now reality.

To my amazing Daughter: Thank you for making me a better person in this life. You are my lion cub and you will roar in this world.

To my Brother and his Family: Thank you for not turning your back on me. Your unconditional love is truly a gift.

To my Best Friend: Thank you for being a man of integrity and compassion. You are my family.

To my Cirque Lodge Family: Thank you for accepting me at my lowest and then building me up to the man I am today. I love and respect every single one of you.

To my Friends and Extended Family: I want to recognize you and say how much your supportive words of encouragement for my recovery journey has meant to me these past eight years. Thank you for the love and positivity.

To the Publisher of this book: Thank you for your time, energy and willingness to get my project done with dignity and professionalism. Now *your* story needs to be heard.

To my Lord and Savior, I want to give everything. None of this would have been possible without Your love, forgiveness, and grace.

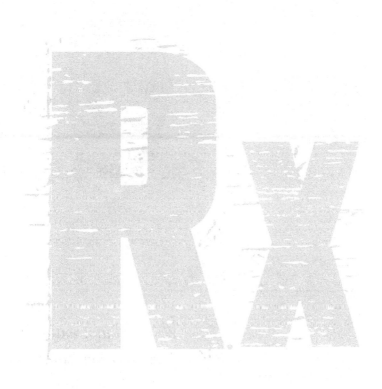

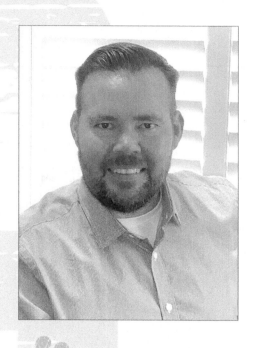

*We're all just walking
each other home.*
—*Ram Dass*

ABOUT THE AUTHOR

Nathan Kruse was born in Lincoln, Nebraska in July of 1977. He traveled the world with his family while growing up in California, Frankfurt, Germany, Florida, and Arizona. Nathan graduated from Orange Park High School in 1996 and then went on to study Golf Course Management and Horticulture at Mundus Institute in Phoenix, Arizona, graduating in 2000. He worked in the Golf industry as a PGA Apprentice until 2002 before selling property and casualty insurance for the next ten years.

In a life-altering decision, Nathan admitted himself into rehab in 2012 at Cirque Lodge in Orem, Utah. After getting sober and starting his Recovery journey,

Part of that journey was opening his own business on *EBay* at the end of 2012 called *JustAppear Retro*, selling men's vintage clothing, footwear, and accessories. He has found much enjoyment and freedom finding used and thrown away items to rehabilitate and sell to his customers, giving those items a second chance to live too.

Nathan has experienced many miracles while in long-term Recovery like becoming engaged to Lizzy, the birth of their daughter Josie in 2018, and rebuilding strong relationships with family and wonderful friends.

Also, in 2018, Nathan received his Certified Peer Support Specialist designation from the Utah Department of Mental Health and Substance Abuse.

Nathan is now using other platforms to share his passion for Recovery like his Podcast, audiobook, and Vlog. You can follow Nathan's journey and find many helpful resources: www.TheRecoveryRx.com.

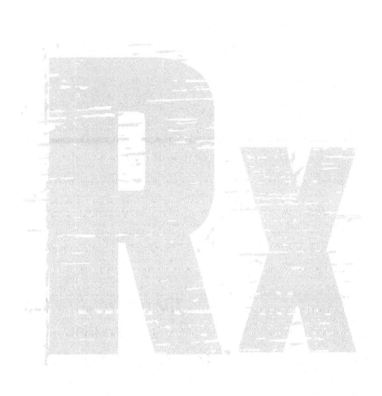

THE END . . . OR THE BEGINNING

*The righteous are bold
as a lion.*

—Proverbs 28: 1